COLOR ATLAS OF INFECTIVE ENDOCARDITIS

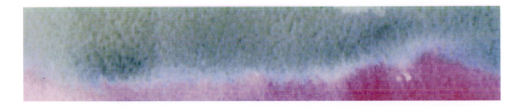

COLOR ATLAS OF INFECTIVE ENDOCARDITIS

David R. Ramsdale BSc, MB ChB, FRCP, MD

Consultant Cardiologist, The Cardiothoracic Centre
Liverpool, UK

With 231 Figures including 159 in Color

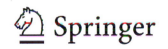

Springer

David R. Ramsdale BSc, MB ChB, FRCP, MD
The Cardiothoracic Centre, Liverpool, UK

British Library Cataloguing in Publication Data
Ramsdale, David R.
   Color atlas of infective endocarditis
   1. Infective endocarditis – Atlases
   I. Title
   66.1'1
ISBN 1852339373

Library of Congress Control Number: 2005923775

ISBN-10: 1-85233-937-3   e-ISBN 1-84628-136-9
ISBN-13: 9781852339371

Printed on acid-free paper

Printed in Singapore

9 8 7 6 5 4 3 2 1

Springer Science+Business Media
springeronline.com

This book is dedicated to Drs Geoffrey Wade and Derek Rowlands, who first introduced me to clinical cardiology and electrocardiography at Manchester University Medical School, and to Drs Colin Bray and David Bennett at Wythenshawe Hospital for the time, training and encouragement they gave to me as their research fellow. Their extraordinary knowledge as well as their great love and dedication to the specialty of cardiology were an inspiration to me.

"We shall never learn to feel and respect our real calling and destiny, unless we have taught ourselves to consider every thing as moonshine, compared with the education of the heart"

—J. G. Lockhart (August 1825), quoted in Lockhart's *Life of Sir Walter Scott*, vol. 6 (1837), ch. 2.

FOREWORD

Infective endocarditis, a dreaded complication of acquired valvular and congenital heart disease, has long been a source of fascination and a challenge to physicians, microbiologists and cardiac surgeons. Despite the landmark development of antibiotic therapy in the 1950s that, for the first time, offered the possibility of cure and the subsequent introduction of cardiac surgery and improved microbiological and imaging techniques, mortality remains high, diagnosis is often difficult and, arguably, many cases could be prevented. With an annual incidence in the United Kingdom of under 1000 cases per year, few cardiologists will have great experience of endocarditis, but it is a condition that requires clinical judgement of the highest order and a multi-disciplinary approach if complications and mortality are to be minimised.

David Ramsdale has a particular interest in and long experience of endocarditis. This book is the culmination of that experience combined with an exhaustive review of the literature carried out during his leadership of a project, on behalf of the British Cardiac Society, to develop guidance on its diagnosis and management. Entitled a *Color Atlas of Infective Endocarditis* because of the large number of superb clinical photographs, many from his own practice, the scope of this monograph far exceeds that of a comprehensive collection of illustrations of the protean manifestations of this disease. Dr Ramsdale has provided us with an authoritative textbook on the contemporary approach to the prevention, diagnosis and management of infective endocarditis. It will provide a valuable source of learning and reference for students, microbiologists, sonographers, dentists, and physicians of all specialties.

Nicholas Brooks
Manchester
July 2005

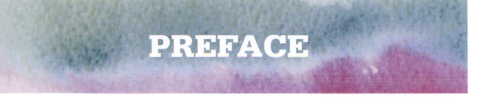

PREFACE

Infective endocarditis is a life-threatening disease with substantial morbidity and mortality (20% or more) despite improved techniques to aid diagnosis and modern antibiotics and surgical therapies. It affects individuals with underlying structural cardiac defects who develop bacteremia, often as a result of dental, gastrointestinal, genitourinary, respiratory, or cardiac invasive/surgical procedures. Most organ systems can be involved and the manner in which infective endocarditis may present to doctors in a variety of specialties demands that they be made aware of infective endocarditis as a potential diagnosis warranting prompt specialist investigation and treatment.

This illustrated book aims to present the clinical manifestations—both cardiac and extracardiac, the diagnostic techniques currently used in clinical practice, the range of microorganisms that are responsible, and the clinical scenarios that are often associated with initiating bacteremia. The guidelines for prophylactic antibiotic therapy to prevent infective endocarditis following dental or invasive/surgical procedures and the medical treatment indicated for both native and prosthetic valve endocarditis are presented in detail. Finally, the indications, timing, and outcome of cardiac surgical intervention and prognosis are discussed.

ACKNOWLEDGMENTS

I acknowledge the expert advice of several colleagues with whom I worked in developing Guidelines for the Management of Infective Endocarditis in Adults on behalf of the Clinical Practice Committee of the British Cardiac Society. These include: Consultant Microbiologists Professor Tom Elliott and Dr Paul Wright; Consultant Cardiothoracic Surgeon Mr Brian Fabri; Specialist Cardiology Registrar Dr Nick Palmer; Consultant Cardiac Anaesthetist Dr Peter Wallace; Consultant Cardiologist Dr Petros Nihoyoannoupolus; and Professor of Paediatric Dentistry, Graham Roberts. Their opinions and advice are truly valued.

I greatly appreciate the generosity of several friends and clinical colleagues who have provided illustrations for the book. These include Consultant Cardiologists Dr David Roberts, Victoria Hospital, Blackpool, UK; Dr Chris Bellamy, Glan Clywd Hospital, Wales, UK; Dr Brad Munt and Dr Robert Moss, St Paul's Hospital, Vancouver, BC, Canada; Dr Nick Newall, Arrowe Park Hospital, Wirral, UK; Dr Peter Schofield, Papworth Hospital, Cambridgeshire, UK; Dr Syamkumar Divakaramenon, Medical College Hospital, Calicut, Kerala, India; Dr Bogdan Marcu, Hospital of Saint Raphael-Yale University, New Haven, CT, USA; Dr Lindsay Morrison, Dr Serge Osula, and Dr Richard Charles, The Cardiothoracic Centre, Liverpool, UK; Specialist registrars in Cardiology, Dr Malcolm Burgess and Dr. Elved Roberts, The Cardiothoracic Centre, Liverpool, UK; Consultant Cardiothoracic Surgeons Mr Niraj Mediratta, Mr Walid Dihmis, Mr John Chalmers, Mr Mark Pullan, Mr Aung Oo, and Mr Abbas Rashid, The Cardiothoracic Centre, Liverpool, UK; Professor John Pepper, Royal Brompton Hospital, London, UK; Specialist registrars in Cardiothoracic Surgery Dr Joanna Chikwe and Dr J. Barnard, Royal Brompton Hospital, London, UK; Consultant Cardiothoracic Anaesthetists Dr Nigel Scawn and Dr Mike Desmond, The Cardiothoracic Centre, Liverpool, UK; Consultant in Infectious Diseases Dr Nick Beeching, Royal Liverpool University Hospital, Liverpool, UK; Consultant Pathologists Dr Hani Zakhour, Arrowe Park Hospital, Wirral, UK, Dr John Gosney, Royal Liverpool University Hospital, Liverpool, UK, and Dr Mary Sheppard, Royal Brompton Hospital, London, UK; Consultant Microbiologists Professor Martin Altwegg, University of Zurich, Switzerland, Dr Lisa Grech, Royal Hallamshire Hospital, Sheffield, UK, Dr John Cunniffe, Arrowe Park Hospital, Wirral, UK, and Dr Mike Rothburn, Aintree Hospital, Liverpool, UK; Consultant Radiologists, Dr Hilary Fewins and Dr John Holemans, The Cardiothoracic Centre, Liverpool, UK; Consultant Neuroradiologist Dr Sacha Niven, Walton Centre for Neurology, Liverpool, UK. Consultant Dental Surgeon Mr Phil Hardy, Liverpool University Dental School, Liverpool, UK; Consultant Dermatologist Dr Graham Sharpe, Royal Liverpool University Hospital, Liverpool, UK; Consultant Opthalmologist, Mr Simon Harding, St Paul's Eye Hospital, Liverpool, UK; Echocardiographers Janet Beukers, Jackie Rolt, Sandra Belchambers, and Amanda Christopher, The Cardiothoracic Centre, Liverpool, UK; and Medical photographers, Mr Phil Rooney, Aintree Hospital, Liverpool, UK and Ms Jackie Hyland, Alder Hey Hospital, Liverpool, UK.

I am also grateful to several other international colleagues for their generosity in allowing me to use their wonderful illustrations. These include Dr Charlie Goldberg,

University of California San Diego, USA; Dr Josh Fierer, Dr Frederick Chen; Dr Hubert Lepidi, Consultant Pathologist, Université de la Mediterranée, Marseille, France; Professor Didier Raoult, Marseille School of Medicine and Director of Clinical Microbiology Laboratories, University Hospitals of Marseille, France; Professor Tomas Freiberger, Centre of Cardiovascular Surgery and Transplantation, Brno, Czech Republic; Dr John E. Moore and Dr B. Cherie Moore, Clinical Scientists, Northern Ireland Public Health Laboratory, Department of Bacteriology, Belfast City Hospital, Northern Ireland.

Finally, I appreciate the personal efforts and technical expertise of all at Springer, and in particular Mr Grant Weston, the commissioning editor, Hannah Wilson, Mr Weston's editorial assistant, and Ms Lesley Poliner, Senior Production Editor, for their conscientious help in coordinating much of the work involved in production.

CONTENTS

CHAPTER 1

Incidence and Pathogenesis

INCIDENCE

Infective endocarditis (IE) is uncommon. The yearly incidence reported in developed countries ranges between 1.8 and 6.2 per 100 000 of the population [1–5]. However, these estimates may be imprecise for a variety of reasons. Although it affects neonates [6,7], infants [8], children [9,10], young adults, and pregnant women [11], the incidence increases after 30 years of age and exceeds 10 per 100 000 for people aged over 50 years [12]. It is a life-threatening disease with a substantial in-hospital morbidity and mortality (approximately 20%) despite improved techniques to aid diagnosis and modern antibiotics and surgical therapies [13]. One-year mortality approaches 40% [14]. Prosthetic valve endocarditis (PVE), although uncommon (0.1–2.3% per patient year) carries an even higher mortality rate [15–17] and prevention of IE is therefore extremely important [18].

ETIOLOGY AND PATHOGENESIS

Infective endocarditis predominantly affects individuals with underlying structural cardiac defects who develop bacteremia with microorganisms likely to cause endocarditis [19]. The incidence and risk of IE in such patients following cardiac surgical and interventional procedures

has been reviewed in the literature [20,21]. Experimental studies suggest that endothelial damage leads to platelet and fibrin deposition and thus a nonbacterial thrombotic endocardial lesion [22,23]. If bacteremia then occurs, for example as a result of a surgical or dental procedure or instrumentation involving mucosal surfaces contaminated by microorganisms, bacteria settle on the damaged or abnormal heart valves or on the endocardium close to anatomic defects resulting in endocarditis or endarteritis. Valvular and congenital cardiac abnormalities, especially those that result in abnormal high-velocity jets, can damage the endothelial surface and predispose to the formation of a potential site for an infective endocardial lesion [24,25] and the pathologic hallmark of endocarditis— infective vegetations (Figure 1.1), which are composed of masses of organisms enmeshed with fibrin, platelets, and variable inflammatory cell infiltrate (Figures 1.2–1.4) [26]. Thus, in patent ductus arteriosus, vegetations usually occur on the pulmonary artery, at the site where the jet of blood from the aorta hits the pulmonary artery through the ductus. In mitral regurgitation, vegetations occur on the atrial aspect of the mitral valve and in aortic regurgitation on the ventricular aspect of the aortic valve. Progressive, uncontrolled infection leads to intracardiac abscess formation, valvular perforation, destruction, and dehiscence causing regurgitation, fistula, and false aneurysm formation as well as devastating embolic and vasculitic complications.

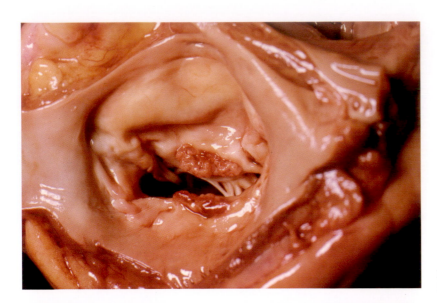

FIGURE 1.1 Large vegetations on the mitral valve in a patient with *Staphylococcus aureus* endocarditis.

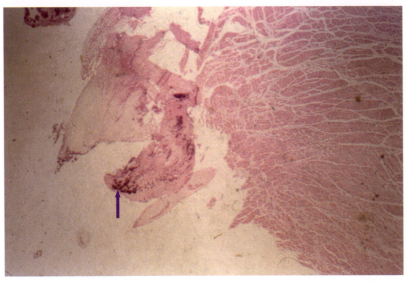

FIGURE 1.2 Histopathology of vegetations containing bacterial colonies (arrow). Courtesy of Dr Hani Zakhour.

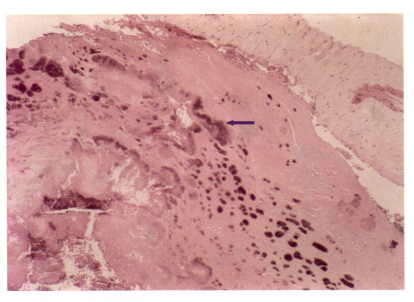

FIGURE 1.3 High-power magnification of vegetations showing bacterial colonies (arrow). Courtesy of Dr Hani Zakhour.

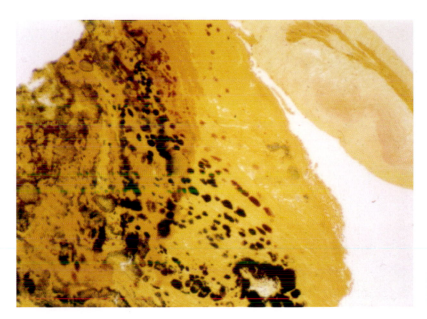

FIGURE 1.4 Histopathology of vegetations showing bacterial colonies stained black. Courtesy of Dr Hani Zakhour.

PATIENTS AT RISK

Currently, patients with prosthetic cardiac valves, users of illicit intravenous (IV) drugs, and patients with mitral valve prolapse or other nonrheumatic heart disease (e.g.

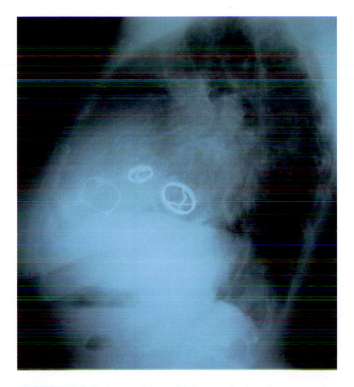

FIGURE 1.5 Patients with multiple prosthetic valves are at increased risk of infective endocarditis. Chest X-ray—left lateral.

congenital heart disease, bicuspid aortic valves), rather than those with rheumatic heart disease, account for the majority of cases of IE, although rheumatic heart disease is still responsible for approximately 40–50% of cases [19,27–31] (Figures 1.5–1.9). Such patients are at increased risk when undergoing invasive procedures. Elderly patients, chronic alcoholics, patients with chronic inflammatory bowel disease, poor dental hygiene, or on chronic hemodialysis, as well as those with diabetes mellitus and those on immunosuppressives are at increased risk of IE [5,32–44]. Left-sided cardiac structures are most commonly affected (85% of cases)—isolated aortic lesions in 55–60%, isolated mitral lesions in 25–30%, and mitral and aortic lesions in 15% of cases. Right-sided IE accounts for 10–15% of cases.

Table 1.1 shows the causes of bacteremia that are responsible for IE and the predominant pathogens that are responsible.

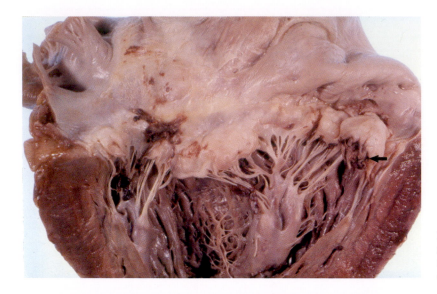

FIGURE 1.6 Patients with mitral valve prolapse and mitral regurgitation are more prone to infective endocarditis. Vegetations can be seen on the leaflets and chordae (arrow). Courtesy of Dr John Gosney.

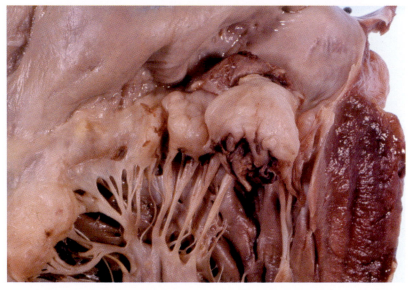

FIGURE 1.7 Large mobile vegetations on this myxomatous prolapsing mitral valve were associated with severe mitral regurgitation and ruptured chordae. This 65-year-old man with *Staphylococcus aureus* endocarditis died of a large cerebral abscess. Courtesy of Dr John Gosney.

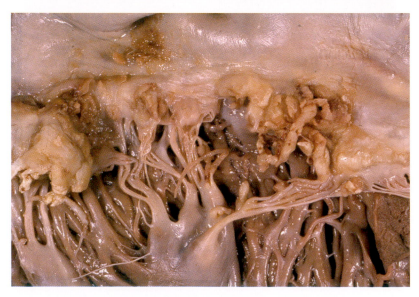

FIGURE 1.8 Large vegetations on a myxomatous mitral valve again associated with severe mitral regurgitation and ruptured chordae. Courtesy of Dr John Gosney.

TABLE 1.1 Causes of Bacteremia Responsible for Infective Endocarditis [45]

Cause	Percent of cases	Predominant pathogen
Dental procedures	20	Penicillin-sensitive viridans streptococci[a] [46–49]
Respiratory tract infection Oropharyngeal surgery Respiratory tract surgery	<5	*Streptococcus pneumoniae*[b] [50–54] *Haemophilus* spp.
Gastrointestinal infectious diseases Gastrointestinal tumors [55] Gastrointestinal tract, therapeutic interventions [60–61] Gallbladder disease [62] Inflammatory bowel disease [63–66]	10–15	Enterococci *Streptococcus bovis* [56–59] [72–75] Gram-negative aerobic bacilli Staphylococci
Urosepsis [67] Urological interventions	5–10	Enterococci [68–71] Gram-negative aerobic bacilli *Staphylococcus aureus*
Gynecological infections Gynecological interventions	1–5	Streptococci Enterococci
Pacemaker implantation/infection (TV) [76,77]		*Staphylococcus epidermidis/S. aureus*

Valvular heart surgery:
  early
 	
  late
		
		Staphylococcus aureus
		Staphylococcus epidermidis
		Staphylococcus aureus, Staphylococcus epidermidis
		Viridans streptococci
		Any organism

Other Dermatological conditions [78–81] Wound infections Skin injuries/burns [82,83] Osteomyelitis [84,85] Intravascular catheters[c] [86–88] Chronic hemodialysis Portosystemic stent shunt [91] IV drug abuse[d] [92–94] Cardiac surgery Ventriculo-atrial shunt [95]	 10–15 10	 *Staphylococcus aureus* *Staphylococcus epidermidis* Gram-negative aerobic bacilli Fungi [89,90]

[a]Viridans streptococci (alpha hemolytic) comprise *S. bovis; S. mutans* (10%); *S. mitis* (25%)—includes *S. sanguis; S. anginosus* (5%)—formerly *S. milleri* group—includes *S. intermedius* [96–98].
[b] *Streptococcus pneumoniae* is infrequent [99,100].
[c]IV lines in patients after valve replacement are important potential causes of IE.
[d] *Staphylococcus aureus* (60%); streptococci and enterococci (20%); Gram-negative aerobic bacilli (10%); fungi (5%).

A wide variety of other microorganisms have been reported to cause IE including: *Neisseria gonorrhoeae* [101–103], *N. meningitidis* [104,105]; HACEK Gram-negative bacilli [106–111]; *Pseudomonas aeruginosa,* [112,113], *P. mendocina* [114]; *Listeria* [115–121]; diphtheroids [122]; *Spirillum* [123]; *Brucella* [124]; *Mycoplasma pneumoniae* [125,126]; *Coxiella burnetii* [127]; *Chlamydia* [128–131]; *Bartonella* [132]; *Salmonella* [133–135]; *Pasteurella* [136,137]; *Yersinia* [138]; *Nocardia* [139]; *Tropheryma whipplei* [140–143]; *Lactobacillus* [144,145]; *Clostridium* [146,147]; *Legionella* [148–150]; *Mycobacterium tuberculosis* [151]; *Rothia dentocarios* [152]; *Erysipelothrix rhusiopathiae* [153]; *Gemella* [154,155]; *Histoplasma* [156]; *Serratia* [157]; *Moraxella* [158]; *Actinomycosis* [159]; *Streptomyces* [160]; group B streptococci [161].

For further references relevant to this section see website: www.bcs.com.

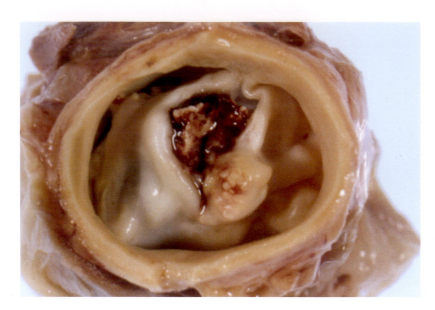

FIGURE 1.9 The large vegetations on this bicuspid aortic valve were due to viridans streptococci. The crusted white nodule on the right is a mass of collagenous fibrosis with calcification. The vegetation virtually occludes the orifice. Courtesy of Dr John Gosney.

REFERENCES

1. van der Meer JT, Thompson J, Valkenburg HA, Michel MF. Epidemiology of bacterial endocarditis in the Netherlands. 1. Patient characteristics. Arch Intern Med 1992;152:1863–1868.

2. Delahaye F, Goulet V, Lacassin F, et al. Epidemiology of infective endocarditis in France in 1991. Arch Mal Coeur 1993;86(Suppl 12):180–186.

3. Horstkotte D, Piper C. Endocarditis. In: Acar J, Bodnar E, eds. Textbook of Acquired Heart Valve Disease, vol. II. London: ICR Publishers; 1995:596–677.

4. Karchmer AW. Infective endocarditis. Braunwald's Heart Disease, 5th edn, vol. 2. Philadelphia: WB Saunders; 1997:1077–1104.

5. Mylonakis E, Calderwood SB. Infective endocarditis in adults. N Engl J Med 2001;345:1318–1330.

6. Mecrow IK, Ladusans EJ. Infective endocarditis in newborn infants with structurally normal hearts. Acta Paediatr 1994;83:35–39.

7. O'Callaghan C, McDougall P. Infective endocarditis in neonates. Arch Dis Child 1988;63:53–57.

8. Lorber A, Luder AS, Dembo L. Acute bacterial endocarditis in early infancy. Int J Cardiol 1987;17:343–345.

9. Fukushige J, Igarashi H, Ueda K. Spectrum of infective endocarditis during infancy and childhood: 20 year review. Pediatr Cardiol 1994;15:127–131.

10. Ferrieri P, Gewitz MH, Gerber MA, et al. Unique features of infective endocarditis in childhood. AHA Scientific Statement. Circulation 2002;105:2115–2127.

11. Dommisse J. Infective endocarditis in pregnancy. A report of 3 cases. S Afr Med J 1988;73:186–187.

12. Selton-Suty C, Hoen B, Grentzinger A, et al. Clinical and bacteriological characteristics of infective endocarditis in the elderly. Heart 1997;77:260–263.

13. Bouza E, Menasalvas A, Munoz P, et al. Infective endocarditis—a prospective study at the end of the twentieth century: new predisposing conditions, new etiologic agents and still a high mortality. Medicine 2001;80:298–307.

14. Cabell CH, Jollis JG, Peterson GE, et al. Changing patient characteristics and the effect on mortality in endocarditis. Arch Intern Med 2002;162:90–94.

15. Schulz R, Werner J, Fuchs B, et al. Clinical outcome and echocardiographic findings of native and prosthetic valve endocarditis in the 1990s. Eur Heart J 1996;17:281–288.

16. Netzer ROM, Zollinger E, Seiler C, et al. Infective endocarditis: clinical spectrum, presentation and outcome. An analysis of 212 cases 1980–1995. Heart 2000;84:25–30.

17. Piper C, Korfer R, Horstkotte D. Prosthetic valve endocarditis. Heart 2001;85:590–593.

18. Leport C, Horstkotte D, Burckhardt D and the Group of Experts of the International Society for Chemotherapy. Antibiotic prophylaxis for infective endocarditis from an international group of experts towards a European consensus. Eur Heart J 1995;16(Suppl B):126–131.

19. McKinsey DS, Ratts TE, Bisno AL. Underlying cardiac lesions in adults with infective endocarditis: The changing spectrum. Am J Med 1987;82:681–688.

20. Michel PL, Acar J. Native cardiac disease predisposing to infective endocarditis. Eur Heart J 1995;16(Suppl B):2–6.

21. de Gevigney G, Pop C, Delahaye JP. The risk of infective endocarditis after cardiac surgical and interventional procedures. Eur Heart J 1995;16:(Suppl B):7–14.

22. Ferguson DJ, McColm AA, Savage TJ, et al. A morphological study of experimental rabbit staphylococcal endocarditis and aortitis. I. Formation and effect of infected and uninfected vegetations on the aorta. Br J Exp Pathol 1986;67:667–678.

23. Ferguson DJP, McColm AA, Ryan DM, Acred P. A morphological study of experimental staphylococcal endocarditis and aortitis. II. Inter-relationship of bacteria, vegetation and cardiovasculature in established infections. Br J Exp Pathol 1986;67:679–686.

24. Lopez JA, Ross RS, Fishbein MC, Siegel RJ. Non bacterial thrombotic endocarditis. A review. Am Heart J 1987;113:773–784.

25. Rodbard S. Blood velocity and endocarditis. Circulation 1963;27:18–25.

26. Livornese IL Jr., Korzeniowski O. Pathogenesis of infective endocarditis. In: Kaye D, ed. Infective Endocarditis, 2nd edn. New York: Raven Press; 1992:19–35.

27. Reisberg BE. Infective endocarditis in the narcotic addict. Prog Cardiovasc Dis 1979;22:193–204.

28. Korzeniowski OM, Kaye D. Infective endocarditis. In: Braunwald E, ed. Heart Disease—A Textbook of Cardiovascular Medicine, 4th edn. Philadelphia: WB Saunders; 1992:1078–1105.

29. Bayliss R, Clarke C, Oakley CM, et al. The microbiology and pathogenesis of infective endocarditis. Br Heart J 1983;50:513–519.

30. Piper C, Horstkotte D, Schulte HD, Schultheib HP. Mitral valve prolapse and infection: a prospective study for risk calculation. Eur Heart J 1996;17(Abstract Suppl):210.

31. Bansal RC. Infective endocarditis. Med Clin North Am 1995;79:1205–1240.

32. Kaye D. Changing pattern of infective endocarditis. Am J Med 1985;78(Suppl 6B):157–162.

33. Buchbinder NA, Roberts WC. Alcoholism: an important but unemphasised factor predisposing to infective endocarditis. Arch Intern Med 1973;132:689–692.

34. Beales IL, Ledson M. Endocarditis in chronic liver disease. Am J Gastroenterol 1994;89:2279.

35. Kreuzpaintner G, Horstkotte D, Heyll A, et al. Increased risk of bacterial endocarditis in inflammatory bowel disease. Am J Med 1992;92:391–395.

36. Cross AS, Steigbigel RJ. Infective endocarditis and access site infections in patients on hemodialysis. Medicine 1976;55:453–466.

37. Dobkin JF, Miller MH, Steigbigel NH. Septicaemia in patients on chronic haemodialysis. Ann Intern Med 1978;88:28–33.

38. Rayfield EJ, Ault MJ, Keusch GT, et al. Infection and diabetes: The case for glucose control. Am J Med 1982;72:439–450.

39. Casey JI, Maturlo S, Albin J, Edberg SC. Comparison of carriage rates of group B streptococcus in diabetic and non-diabetic persons. Am J Epidemiol 1982;116:704–708.

40. Gallagher PG, Watanakunakorn C. Group B streptococcal endocarditis: Report of seven cases and review of the literature, 1962–1985. Rev Infect Dis 1986;8:175–188.

41. Wilkinson NM. Fatal bacterial endocarditis following aortic valve replacement in a patient being treated with methotrexate. J Heart Valve Dis 1999;8:591–592.

42. Hearn CJ, Smedira NG. Pulmonic valve endocarditis after orthotopic liver transplantation. Liver Transpl Surg 1999;5:456–457.

43. Strom BL, Abrutyn E, Berlin JA, et al. Risk factors for infective endocarditis: oral hygiene and non-dental exposure. Circulation 2000;102:2842–2848.

44. Steckelberg JM, Wilson WR. Risk factors for infective endocarditis. Infect Dis Clin North Am 1993;7:9–19.

45. Lacassin F, Hoen B, Leport C, et al. Procedures associated with infective endocarditis in adults. A case control study. Eur Heart J 1995;16:1968–1974.

46. Roberts RB, Krieger AG, Schiller NL, Gross KC. Viridans streptococcal endocarditis: the role of various species including pyridoxal-dependent streptococci. Rev Infect Dis 1979;1:955–966.

47. Coykendall AL. Classification and identification of the viridans streptococci. Clin Microbiol Rev 1989;2:315–328.

48. Harder EJ, Wilkowske CJ, Washington JA 2nd, Geracci JG. *Streptococcus mutans* endocarditis. Ann Intern Med 1974;80:364–368.

49. Stein DS, Nelson KE. Endocarditis due to nutritionally deficient streptococci: therapeutic dilemma. Rev Infect Dis 1987;9:908–916.

50. Gelfand MS, Threlkeld MG. Subacute bacterial endocarditis secondary to *Streptococcus pneumoniae*. Am J Med 1992;93:91–93.

51. Ugolini V, Pacifico A, Smitherman TC, Mackowiak PA. Pneumococcal endocarditis update: analysis of 10 cases diagnosed between 1974 and 1984. Am Heart J 1986;112:813–819.

52. Powderly WG, Stanley SL, Medoff G. Pneumococcal endocarditis: report of a series and review of the literature. Rev Infect Dis 1986;8:786–791.

53. Sands M, Brown RB, Ryczak M, Hamilton W. *Streptococcus pneumoniae* endocarditis. South Med J 1987;80:780–782.

54. Lindberg J, Fangel S. Recurrent endocarditis caused by *Streptococcus pneumoniae*. Scand J Infect Dis 1999;31:409–410.

55. Marshall JB, Gerhardt DC. Polyposis coli presenting with *Streptococcus bovis* endocarditis. Am J Gastroenterol 1981;75:314–316.

56. Kupferwasser I, Darius H, Muller AM, et al. Clinical and morphological characteristics in *Streptococcus bovis* endocarditis: a comparison with other causative microorganisms in 177 cases. Heart 1998;80:276–280.

57. Seglenieks A, Black RB. *Streptococcus bovis* and its association with bowel cancer. Aust N Z J Surg 1998;68:542–543.

58. Ben-Haim SA, Nechmad M, Edoute Y, et al. Colonic villous adenoma, polyp and leiomyoma presenting with *Streptococcus bovis* endocarditis. Am Heart J 1988;115:192–195.

59. Zuccollo R, Boyd RV. *Streptococcus bovis* endocarditis and carcinoma of the colon. Br J Clin Pract 1987;41:1022–1023.

60. Wong A, Rosenstein AH, Rutherford RE, James SP. Bacterial endocarditis following endoscopic variceal sclerotherapy. J Clin Gastroenterol 1997;24:90–91.

61. Baskin G. Prosthetic endocarditis after endoscopic variceal sclerotherapy: a failure of antibiotic prophylaxis. Am J Gastroenterol 1989;84:311–312.

62. Bortolotto LA, Mansur AJ, Grinberg M, et al. Infective endocarditis related to acute cholecystitis. Thorac Cardiovasc Surg 1988;36:237–238.

63. Kreuzpaintner G, Horstkotte D, Heyll A, et al. Increased risk of bacterial endocarditis in inflammatory bowel disease. Am J Med 1992;92:391–395.

64. Nicholls DP, Stanford CF. Infective endocarditis due to ulcerative colitis. Ulster Med J 1991;60:114–116.

65. Wong JS. Infective endocarditis in Crohn's disease. Br Heart J 1989;62:163–164.

66. Ward RL. Endocarditis complicating ulcerative colitis. Gastroenterology 1977;73:1189–1190.

67. Hoffman MA, Steele G, Yalla S. Acute bacterial endocarditis secondary to prostatic abscess. J Urol 2000;163:245.

68. Bisno AL, Dismukes WE, Durack DT, et al. Antimicrobial treatment of infective endocarditis due to viridans streptococci, enterococci and staphylococci. JAMA 1989;261:1471–1477.

69. Jones BL, Ludlam HA, Brown DF. High dose ampicillin for the treatment of high-level aminoglycoside resistant enterococcal endocarditis. J Antimicrob Chemother 1994;33:891–892.

70. Mandell GL, Kaye D, Levison ME, Hook EW. Enterococcal endocarditis: An analysis of 38 patients observed at the New York Hospital-Cornell Medical Center. Arch Intern Med 1970;125:258–264.

71. Maki DG, Agger WA. Enterococcal bacteremia: clinical features, the risk of endocarditis and management. Medicine 1988;67:248–269.

72. Moellering RC Jr, Watson BK, Kunz LJ. Endocarditis due to group D streptococci. Comparison of disease caused by *Streptococcus bovis* with that produced by enterococci. Am J Med 1974;57:239–250.

73. Leport C, Bure A, Leport J, Vilde JL. Incidence of colonic lesions in *Streptococcus bovis* and enterococcal endocarditis. Lancet 1987;i:748.

74. Emiliani VJ, Chodos JE, Comer GM, et al. *Streptococcus bovis* brain abscess associated with an occult colonic villous adenoma. Am J Gastroenterol 1990;85:78–80.

75. Wiseman A, Rene P, Crelinstein GL. *Streptococcus agalactiae* endocarditis: an association with villous adenomas of the large intestine. Ann Intern Med 1985;103:893–894.

76. Arber N, Pras E, Copperman Y, et al. Pacemaker endocarditis. Report of 44 cases and review of the literature. Medicine 1994;73:299–305.

77. Vlay SC. Prevention of bacterial endocarditis in patients with permanent pacemakers and automatic internal cardioverter defibrillators. Am Heart J 1990;120:1490–1492.

78. Kobayashi H, Sugiuchi R, Tabata N, et al. Guess what! Acute infective endocarditis with Janeway lesions in a patient with atopic dermatitis. Eur J Dermatol 1999;9:239–240.

79. Grabczynska SA, Cerio R. Infective endocarditis associated with atopic eczema. Br J Dermatol 1999;140:1193–1194.

80. Ostlere LS, Akhras F, Langtry JA, Staughton RC. Generalized pustular psoriasis associated with bacterial endocarditis of the anterior papillary muscle. Br J Dermatol 1992;127:187–188.

81. Pike MG, Warner JO. Atopic dermatitis complicated by acute bacterial endocarditis. Acta Paediatr Scand 1989;78:463–464.

82. Gowda TK, Sriprasad S, Korath MP, Jagadeesan K. Right ventricular mural infective endocarditis in a patient with burns. J Assoc Physicians India 1992;40:52–54.

83. Hassan IJ, Carmichael A. Endocarditis following skin procedures. J Infect 1993;27:341–342.

84. Speechly-Dick ME, Swanton RH. Osteomyelitis and infective endocarditis. Postgrad Med J 1994;70:885–890.

85. Speechly-Dick ME, Vaux EC, Swanton RH. A case of osteomyelitis secondary to endocarditis. Br Heart J 1994;72:298.

86. Weidmann B, Hanseler T, Jimenez C, Niederle N. Tricuspid endocarditis induced by implantable venous access. J Clin Oncol 1994;12:1103–1105.

87. Bernardin G, Milhaud D, Roger PM, et al. Swan-Ganz catheter-related pulmonary valve infective endocarditis: a case report. Intensive Care Med 1994;20:142–144.

88. Kaye GC, Rodgers H, Smith DR, Turney J. Bacterial endocarditis of the tricuspid valve after insertion of a central venous catheter. Br J Clin Pract 1990;44:762–763.

89. Rubinstein E, Lang R. Fungal endocarditis. Eur Heart J 1995;16(Suppl B):84–89.

90. Rubinstein E, Noriega ER, Simberkoff MS, Holzman R, Rahal Jr JJ. Fungal endocarditis: analysis of 24 cases and review of the literature. Medicine 1975;54:331–344.

91. Finkielman JD, Gimenez M, Pietrangelo C, Blanco MV. Endocarditis as a complication of a transjugular intrahepatic portosystemic stent-shunt. Clin Infect Dis 1996;22:385–386.

92. Julander I. Staphylococcal septicaemia and endocarditis in 80 drug addicts. Aspects on epidemiology, clinical and laboratory findings and prognosis. Scand J Infect Dis 1983;41(Suppl):49–55.

93. Levine DP, Crane LR, Zervos MJ. Bacteremia in narcotic addicts at the Detroit Medical Center. II. Infectious endocarditis: A prospective comparative study. Rev Infect Dis 1986;8:374–396.

94. Eichacker PQ, Miller K, Robbins M, et al. Echocardiographic evaluation of heart valves in IV drug abusers without a previous history of endocarditis. Clin Res 1984;32:670A.

95. Bellamy CM, Roberts DH, Ramsdale DR. Ventriculo-atrial shunt causing tricuspid endocarditis: its percutaneous removal. Int J Cardiol 1990;28:260–262.

96. Molina JM, Leport C, Bure A, et al. Clinical and bacterial features of infections caused by *Streptococcus milleri*. Scand J Infect Dis 1991;23:659–692.

97. Ullman RF, Miller SJ, Strampfer MJ, Cunha BA. *Streptococcus mutans* endocarditis: report of three cases and review of the literature. Heart Lung 1988;17:209–212.

98. Boenning DA, Nelson LP, Campos JM. Relatively penicillin-resistant *Streptococcus sanguis* endocarditis in an adolescent. Pediatr Infect Dis J 1988;7:205–207.

99. Endara A, Corkerton MA, Diqer AM, Neal AJ, Kang D. Pneumococcal aortic valve endocarditis causing aortopulmonary artery fistula. Ann Thorac Surg 2001;72:1737–1738.

100. Siegel M, Timpane J. Penicillin-resistant *Streptococcus pneumoniae* endocarditis: a case report and review. Clin Infect Dis 2001;32:972–974.

101. Wall TC, Peyton RB, Corey GR. Gonococcal endocarditis: a new look at an old disease. Medicine 1989;68:375–380.

102. Owens JE, Kelchak JA. Gonococcal endocarditis: report of a case and review of the literature. J S C Med Assoc 1990;86: 93–96.

103. Jackman JD Jr, Glamann DB. Gonococcal endocarditis: twenty-five year experience. Am J Med Sci 1991;301:221–230.

104. Gunn J, Gaw A, Trueman AM. A case of meningococcal endocarditis. Eur Heart J 1992;13:1004–1005.

105. Candrick J, Segasothym M, Wheaton G, et al. Meningococcal endocarditis in a patient with rheumatic heart disease. Aust N Z J Med 1999;29:749–750.

106. Lynn DJ, Kane JG, Parker RH. *Haemophilus parainfluenzae* and *influenzae* endocarditis: a review of forty cases. Medicine 1977;56:115–128.

107. Ellner JJ, Rosenthal MS, Lerner PI, McHenry MC. Infective endocarditis caused by slow-growing, fastidious, Gram-negative bacteria. Medicine 1979;58:145–158.

108. Schack SH, Smith PW, Penn RG, Rapoport JM. Endocarditis caused by *Actinobacillus actinomycetemcomitans*. J Clin Microbiol 1984;20:579–581.

109. Lane T, MacGregor RR, Wright D, Hollander J. *Cardiobacterium hominis*: an elusive cause of endocarditis. J Infect Dis 1983;6:75–80.

110. Decker MD, Graham BS, Hunter ER, Liebowitz SM. Endocarditis and infections of intravascular devices due to *Eikenella corrodens*. Am J Med Sci 1986;292:209–212.

111. Jenny DB, Letendre PW, Iverson G. Endocarditis due to *Kingella* species. Rev Infect Dis 1988;10:1065–1066.

112. Cohen PS, Maguire JH, Weinstein L. Infective endocarditis caused by gram-negative bacteria: a review of the literature. Prog Cardiovasc Dis 1980;22:205–242.

113. Komshian SV, Tablan OC, Palutke W, Reyes MP. Characteristics of left-sided endocarditis due to *Pseudomonas aeruginosa* in the Detroit Medical Center. Rev Infect Dis 1990;12:693–702.

114. Johansen HK, Kjeldsen K, Hoiby N. *Pseudomonas mendocina* as a cause of chronic infective endocarditis in a patient with situs inversus. Clin Microbiol Infect 2001;7:650–652.

115. Carvajal A, Frederiksen W. Fatal endocarditis due to *Listeria monocytogenes*. Rev Infect Dis 1988;10:616–623.

116. Spyrou N, Anderson M, Foale R. Listeria endocarditis: current management and patient outcome—world literature review. Heart 1997;77:380–383.

117. Baddour LM. Listeria endocarditis following coronary artery bypass surgery. Rev Infect Dis 1989;11:669.

118. Castro Cabezas M, Cramer MJ, de Jongh BM, de Maat CE. *Listeria monocytogenes* endocarditis in a patient with an aortic prosthetic valve. Neth J Med 1996;48:15–17.

119. Johnston PW, Trouton TG. Dietary precautions and listeria endocarditis? Heart 1998;79:206.

120. Alonso J, Revuelta JM, Marce L, et al. Successful surgical treatment of a case of *Listeria monocytogenes* endocarditis. J Cardiovasc Surg 1988;29:140–142.

121. Gallagher PG, Watanakunakorn C. *Listeria monocytogenes* endocarditis: a review of the literature 1950–1986. Scand J Infect Dis 1988;20:359–368.

122. Lindner PS, Hardy DJ, Murphy TF. Endocarditis due to *Corynebacterium pseudodiphtheriticum*. N Y State J Med 1986;86:102–104.

123. McIntosh CS, Vickers PJ, Isaacs AJ. Spirillum endocarditis. Postgrad Med J 1975;51:645–648.

124. Al-Kasab S, al-Fagih MR, al-Yousef S, et al. Brucella infective endocarditis. Successful combined medical and surgical therapy. J Thorac Cardiovasc Surg 1988;95:862–867.

125. Popat K, Barnardo D, Webb-Peploe M. *Mycoplasma pneumoniae* endocarditis. Br Heart J 1980;44:111–112.

126. Cohen JI, Sloss LJ, Kundsin R, Golightly L. Prosthetic valve endocarditis caused by *Mycoplasma hominis*. Am J Med 1989;86:819–821.

127. Stein A, Raoult D. Q fever endocarditis. Eur Heart J 1995;16(Suppl B):19–23.

128. Jones RB, Priest JB, Kuo C. Subacute chlamydial endocarditis. JAMA 1982;247:655–658.

129. Etienne J, Ory D, Thouvenot D, et al. Chlamydial endocarditis: a report of 10 cases. Eur Heart J 1992;13:1422–1426.

130. Norton R, Schepetiuk S, Kok TW. *Chlamydia pneumoniae* pneumonia with endocarditis. Lancet 1995;345:1376–1377.

131. Lamaury I, Sotto A, Le Quellec A, et al. *Chlamydia psittaci* as a cause of lethal bacterial endocarditis. Clin Infect Dis 1993;17:821–822.

132. Baorts E, Payne RM, Slater LN, et al. Culture-negative endocarditis caused by *Bartonella henselae*. J Pediatr 1998;132:1051–1054.

133. Keller LS, Sanders P, Shaw D, Broun MA. Salmonella prosthetic valve (mechanical) endocarditis managed conservatively. Intern Med J 2001;31:364–365.

134. Flannery MT, Le M, Altus P. Endocarditis due to salmonelli. South Med J 2001;94:427–428.

135. Gomez-Moreno J, Moar C, Roman F. Salmonella endocarditis presenting as a cerebral haemorrhage. Eur J Intern Med 2000;11:96–97.

136. Rosenbach KA, Poblete J, Larkin I. Prosthetic valve endocarditis caused by *Pasteurella dagmatis*. South Med J 2001;94:1033–1035.

137. Elsaghier AA, Kibbler CC, Hamilton-Miller JM. *Pasteurella multocida* as an infectious cause of endocarditis. Clin Infect Dis 1998;27:410–411.

138. LeMoal G, Roblot F, Paccalin M, et al. Pacemaker endocarditis due to *Yersinia enterocolitica*. Scand J Infect Dis 2001;33:397.

139. Watson A, French P, Wilson M. *Nocardia asteroides* native valve endocarditis. Clin Infect Dis 2001;32:660–661.

140. Mannaerts HF, Hekker T, Visser CA. A rare case of aortic valve endocarditis caused by *Tropheryma whippelii* with left coronary cusp perforation diagnosed by transoesophageal echocardiography and PCR. Heart 1999;81:217.

141. Fenollar F, Lepidi H, Raoult D. Whipple's endocarditis: review of the literature and comparisons with Q fever, *Bartonella* infection and blood culture-positive endocarditis. Clin Infect Dis 2001;33:1309–1316.

142. Gubler JG, Kuster M, Dutly F, et al. Whipple endocarditis without overt gastrointestinal disease: report of four cases. Ann Intern Med 1999;1341:112–116.

143. Smith MA. Whipple endocarditis without gastrointestinal disease. Ann Intern Med 2000;132:595.

144. Antony S, Dummer S, Stratton C. *Lactobacillus* bacteremia and endocarditis. Clin Infect Dis 1998;26:1483–1484.

145. Atkins MC, Nicolson L, Harrison GA, et al. *Lactobacillus jensenii* prosthetic valve endocarditis. J Infect 1990;21:322–324.

146. Cohen CA, Almeder LM, Israni A, Maslow JN. *Clostridium septicum* endocarditis complicated by aortic-ring abscess and aortitis. Clin Infect Dis 1998;26:495–496.

147. Mendes CM, Oplustil CP, dos Santos TJ, Mady C. *Clostridium perfringens* as a cause of infectious endocarditis in a patient with a vascular prosthesis. Clin Infect Dis 1996;22:866–867.

148. Chen TT, Schapiro JM, Loutit J. Prosthetic valve endocarditis due to *Legionella pneumophila*. J Cardiovasc Surg 1996;37:631–633.

149. Kundsin RB, Walter CW. *Legionella* prosthetic-valve endocarditis. N Engl J Med 1988;319:581.

150. Tompkins LS, Roessler BJ, Redd SC, et al. *Legionella* prosthetic-valve endocarditis. N Engl J Med 1988;318:530–535.

151. Klinger K, Brandli O, Doerfler M, et al. Valvular endocarditis due to *Mycobacterium tuberculosis*. Int J Tuberc Lung Dis 1998;2:435–437.

152. Isaacson JH, Grenko RT. *Rothia dentocariosa* endocarditis complicated by brain abscess. Am J Med 1988;84:352–354.

153. Gorby GL, Peacock JE Jr. *Erysipelothrix rhusiopathiae* endocarditis: microbiologic, epidemiologic and clinical features of an occupational disease. Rev Infect Dis 1988;10:317–325.

154. Samuel L, Bloomfield P, Ross P. *Gemella haemolysans* prosthetic valve endocarditis. Postgrad Med J 1995;71:188.

155. Martin MJ, Wright DA, Jones AR. A case of *Gemella morbillorum* endocarditis. Postgrad Med J 1995;71:188.

156. Wilmshurst PT, Venn GE, Eykyn SJ. *Histoplasma* endocarditis on a stenosed aortic valve presenting as dysphagia and weight loss. Br Heart J 1993;70:565–567.

157. Ena J, Amador C, Parras F, Bouza E. Ciprofloxacin as an effective antibacterial agent in *Serratia* endocarditis. J Infect 1991;22:103–105.

158. Sanyal SK, Wilson N, Twum-Danso K, et al. *Moraxella* endocarditis following balloon angioplasty of aortic coarctation. Am Heart J 1990;119:1421–1423.

159. Lam S, Samraj J, Rahman S, Hilton E. Primary actinomycotic endocarditis: case report and review. Clin Infect Dis 1993;16:481–485.

160. Mossad SB, Tomford JW, Stewart R, Ratliff NB, Hall GS. Case report of *Streptomyces* endocarditis of a prosthetic aortic valve. J Clin Microbiol 1995;33:3335–3337.

161. Gallagher PG, Watanakunakorn C. Group B streptococcal endocarditis: report of seven cases and review of the literature, 1962–1985. Rev Infect Dis 1986;8:175–188.

CHAPTER 2

Clinical Features

CLINICAL MANIFESTATIONS

The clinical manifestations of IE will depend on factors such as the nature of any predisposing condition, the virulence of the responsible organism, and the portal of entry [1].

Patients with acute IE typically present with an accelerated illness including high remitting pyrexia, rigors, and prostration [2,3] (Figure 2.1). It is usually caused by virulent pathogens such as *Staphylococcus aureus* and preexisting valve disease can be minimal. In contrast, those with subacute endocarditis present more insidiously with anorexia, weight loss, fever, chills, myalgia, arthralgia, and fatigue [4,5]. It usually affects patients with major preexisting heart valve defects and is caused by less virulent pathogens such as the viridans streptococci. Unique features occur in childhood [6]. However, there is great variability in the clinical presentation, which is often related to the type of organism responsible and the portal of entry.

The clinical manifestations may be classified as cardiac and extracardiac, although specific features may be found in patients with right-sided IE, PVE, fungal IE, and culture-negative IE (CNE).

CARDIAC

Cardiac manifestations usually dominate the clinical presentation with the presence of new or worsening cardiac murmurs or the development of cardiac failure due to advanced valvular infection and destruction [4,7,8]. Eighty percent of patients present with a murmur whilst 15–20% develop one in hospital [9,10]. Preexisting heart disease is found in 60–75% of cases of left-sided endocarditis but is less common in right-sided disease. The degree of valvular destruction depends on the organism responsible, the duration of infection and its anatomic site. It may consist of ulceration, tear and rupture of mitral or tricuspid chordae tendineae, perforation of the cusps themselves, and even valvular disruption and dehiscence resulting in moderate or severe regurgitation [11] (Figure 2.2). Typically, vegetations occur on the atrial surface of the mitral valve, on the ventricular surface of the aortic valve, distal to a coarctation of the aorta, in the pulmonary artery in association with a patent ductus, and on the right side of a ventricular septal defect. Occasionally all four valves are affected and mural endocarditis occurs [12]. Eustachian valve endocarditis has also been reported [13–16].

Abscesses of the heart are observed in 20–40% of cases, mainly in the aortic valve ring [17–21]. They can spread to surrounding structures such as the aorta, the anterior mitral valve leaflet, and the interventricular septum and can cause a fistula between the two ventricles, between the aorta and left atrium, right atrium or right ventricle, between the left ventricle and the right atrium, and even into the pericardial cavity causing tamponade [19–25]. Rupture of the sinus of Valsalva is usually associated with the development of a continuous murmur, cardiac failure, and a high mortality [26]. Septal abscesses can lead to progressive

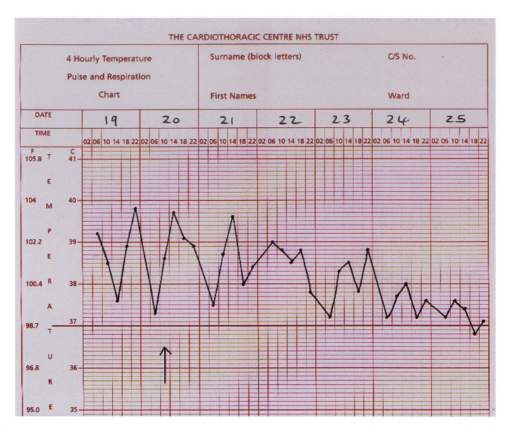

FIGURE 2.1 High remitting pyrexia often associated with rigors is a presenting feature of infective endocarditis. IV antibiotics (arrow) produce a favorable response.

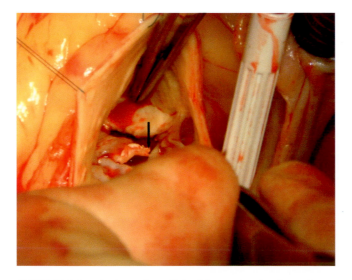

FIGURE 2.2 Infective endocarditis of the aortic valve due to *Streptococcus faecalis* causing detachment of the right coronary cusp (arrow). Courtesy of Mr Walid Dihmis.

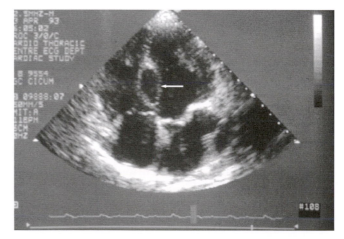

FIGURE 2.3 Abscess of the interventricular septum (arrow) can lead to progressive conduction defects including complete heart block and asystole. Courtesy of Dr L. Morrison.

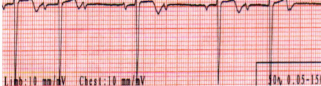

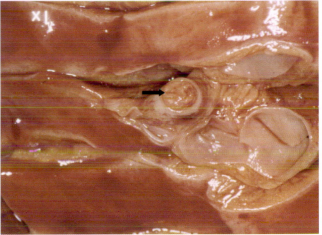

FIGURE 2.4 Conduction disturbances such as complete heart block (as shown here) may occur as a complication of infective endocarditis especially aortic valve endocarditis when infection extends into the interventricular septum (see Figure 2.3).

FIGURE 2.6 Embolization and occlusion of a coronary artery by a large friable vegetation (arrow) from the aortic valve resulted in acute myocardial infarction and death (see Figure 2.7). Courtesy of Dr Hani Zakhour.

conduction defects evidenced by prolongation of the PR interval and leading to complete heart block [23,27] (Figures 2.3 and 2.4). This is more often associated with PVE than with native valve endocarditis (NVE) and native aortic than mitral valve endocarditis. Aortic root abscesses may produce a sinus of Valsalva aneurysm (Figure 2.5) or involve the coronary ostia, and large vegetations can cause valvular obstruction [28,29]. Subaortic aneurysm has been reported [30]. Occasionally, chest pain due to pleurisy, pericarditis or myocardial infarction resulting from coro-

nary arterial emboli are presenting symptoms [31–34] (Figures 2.6–2.10). An inflammatory or septic pericardial effusion is mainly observed in patients with aortic valve endocarditis but pericardial abscess may occur as a result of infection on the mitral valve [19]. Primary involvement of the myocardium occurs with reduction in contractility and ST-T wave abnormalities and ventricular arrhythmias may result (Figures 2.11–2.14). Free wall myocardial abscesses may rupture and cause sudden death [35–37] (Figures 2.15–2.17).

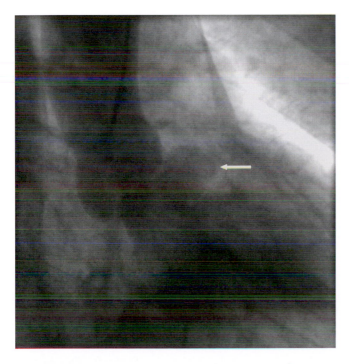

FIGURE 2.5 Aortogram in a 70-year-old man with infective endocarditis of the aortic valve due to viridans streptococci. The illustration shows severe aortic regurgitation and an aneurysm of the sinus of Valsalva (arrow).

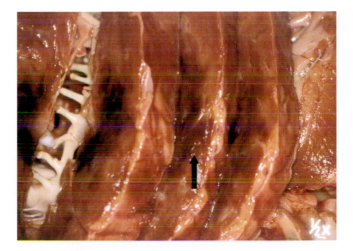

FIGURE 2.7 Myocardial infarction (arrow) following acute coronary occlusion by an embolized vegetation from the aortic valve. Courtesy of Dr Hani Zakhour.

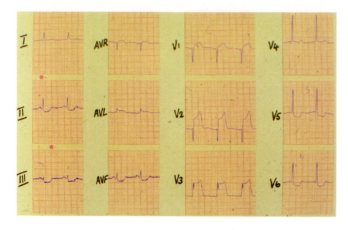

FIGURE 2.8 Twelve-lead ECG showing acute ST-segment elevation in leads V1–V3 due to acute myocardial infarction following a devastating coronary embolus from an aortic valve vegetation.

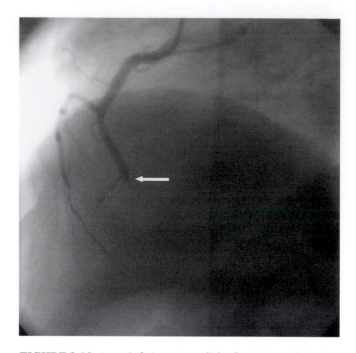

FIGURE 2.10 Acute inferior myocardial infarction may be due to obstruction of the right coronary artery by an embolized vegetation from the aortic valve resulting in total coronary occlusion (arrow), as shown by this right coronary arteriogram.

EXTRACARDIAC

Extracardiac clinical manifestations consist of embolic (13–40%) as well as vasculitic phenomena [33,38,39]—the latter probably being due to immune-complex deposition. Embolic events usually occur early. Focal pain in the flanks or left upper quadrant may be due to embolic infarcts in the kidneys (Figures 2.18–2.21) or spleen (Figures 2.22 and 2.23). Bowel ischemia may be a result of mesenteric embolism. Retinal and peripheral limb emboli may also occur and digital infarction and gangrene may be a feature (Figure 2.24). Splenomegaly is found in 30–50% [17,38,40]; splenic abscesses sometimes occur and splenic rupture can be fatal [41,42]. Abdominal CT or MRI scans appear to be

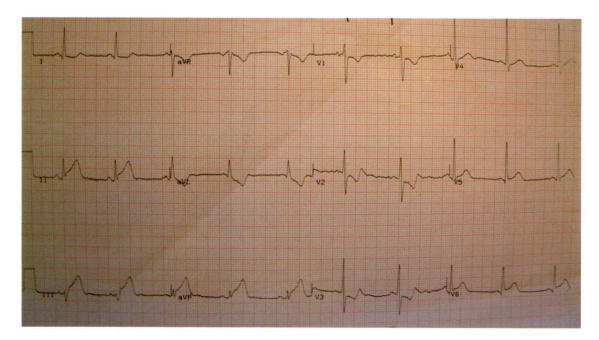

FIGURE 2.9 Twelve-lead ECG showing acute ST-segment elevation in leads II, III, and aVF suggests acute inferior myocardial infarction as a complication of aortic valve endocarditis.

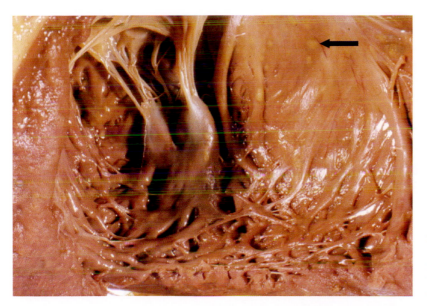

FIGURE 2.11 Myocardial abscesses (arrow) due to *Staphylococcus aureus* endocarditis in a 25-year-old male IV drug abuser dying of septicemia. Abscesses were also found in liver, spleen, and brain. Courtesy of Dr John Gosney.

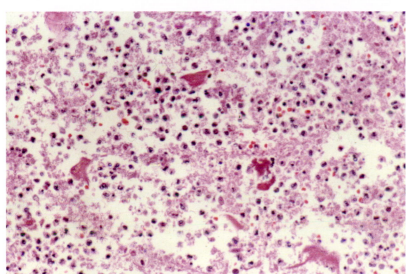

FIGURE 2.12 Histology of the myocardial abscess showing necrotic myocardium, fragmented cardiomyocytes, and an inflammatory response with monocytes, neutrophil leukocytes, and red blood cells. Courtesy of Dr John Gosney.

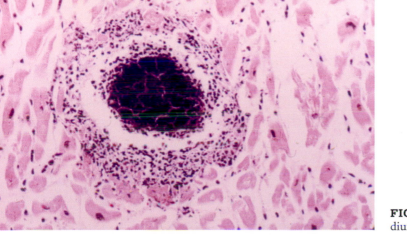

FIGURE 2.13 Focal microabscess in the myocardium due to *Staphylococcus aureus*.

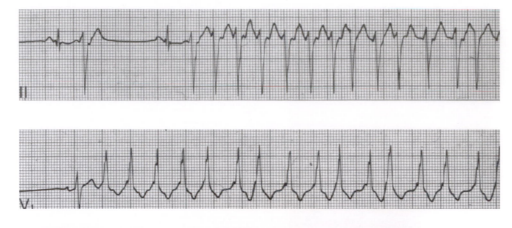

FIGURE 2.14 Direct involvement of the myocardium can cause serious arrhythmias such as ventricular tachycardia.

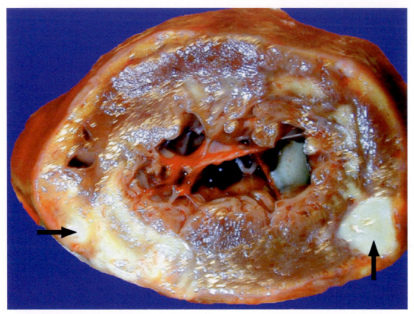

FIGURE 2.15 Large myocardial abscesses (arrows) in the left and right ventricular free wall and interventricular septum in a 53-year-old woman who developed septicemia due to *Staphylococcus aureus* following emergency laparotomy for small bowel obstruction. Five days postoperatively she developed pyrexia, oliguria, hemodynamic instability, peripheral limb infarcts, as well as severe mitral and aortic valve regurgitation. She died in theatre after debridement of an aortic root abscess, homograft replacement of her aortic root, and removal of a mitral valve vegetation.

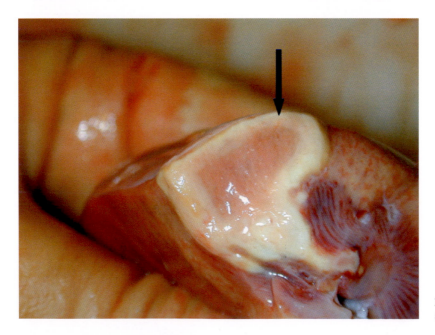

FIGURE 2.16 Renal (arrow), splenic, and cerebral abscesses were found at post-mortem in this patient.

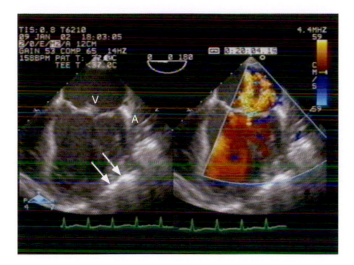

FIGURE 2.17 Her transesophageal echocardiogram demonstrated severe mitral and aortic regurgitation, a 2 cm vegetation (v) on the posterior leaflet of the mitral valve and echodense areas in the interventricular septum (arrows). Figures 2.15–2.17 were kindly provided courtesy of Drs J. Chikwe, J. Barnard, J.R. Pepper, and C. Sheppard. Heart 2004;90:597. Reproduced with permission from the BMJ Publishing Group.

the best diagnostic tests for a splenic hematoma or splenic abscess (Figures 2.25 a and b) and urgent drainage or splenectomy may be necessary.

Neurological manifestations may be the presenting feature [43,44]. These may be headache or any symptoms and signs associated with focal cerebral infarcts (Figures 2.26–2.28), cerebritis or abscess, hemorrhage or mycotic aneurysm, including stroke, drowsiness, confusion, and seizures [45–48]. Subarachnoid and intracerebral hemorrhage are uncommon presenting features. Meningism/meningitis may occur and CSF cultures may be positive [49]. These are particularly serious and life-threatening features with a mortality rate of 40%. A cerebral scan should be performed and in those with cerebral hemorrhage, arteriography or MRI angiogram to look for a mycotic aneurysm (Figure 2.29 a and b). Approximately 3% of all patients with IE develop small aneurysms on the distal branches of the middle, anterior, or posterior cerebral arteries (Figure 2.30). About 65% of these rupture within the first 5 weeks with a high mortality rate (Figure 2.31). Emergency treatment is required to treat or prevent rupture of a mycotic aneurysm or a space-occupying lesion such as a cerebral abscess.

Other vascular or immune-mediated phenomena may occur, including petechiae (20–40%) (on extremities, above clavicles, buccal and palatal mucosa or on palpebral conjunctiva) (Figure 2.32), splinter hemorrhages (5–20%) (Figures 2.33–2.35), retinal hemorrhages, Roth spots (5–10%) (Figure 2.36), painful Osler's nodes (5–15%)

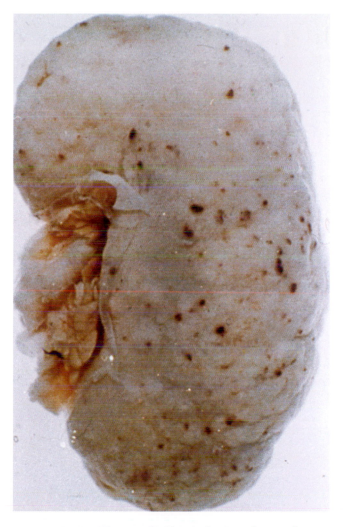

FIGURE 2.18 Diffuse petechial hemorrhages on the capsular surface of the kidney—the "flea-bitten kidney" represents the macroscopic appearance of the focal embolic nephritis that occurs in infective endocarditis.

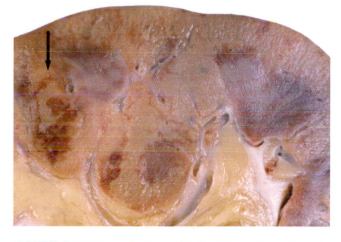

FIGURE 2.19 Hemorrhagic renal infarct (arrow) due to septic emboli in a patient with *Staphylococcus aureus* endocarditis of the aortic and mitral valves. Courtesy of Dr Hani Zakhour.

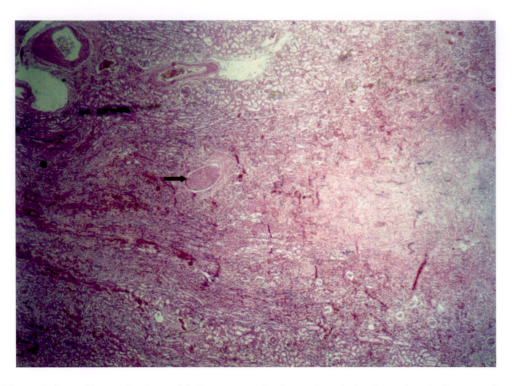

FIGURE 2.20 Histopathology of hemorrhagic renal infarct as a result of a septic embolus (arrow) occluding a renal artery. Courtesy of Dr Hani Zakhour.

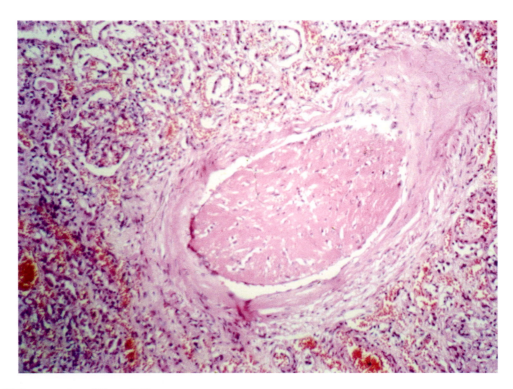

FIGURE 2.21 High power view of Figure 2.20.

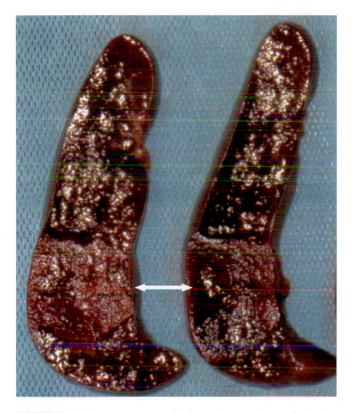

FIGURE 2.22 Cross-section of spleen showing hemorrhagic infarct (arrow) due to systemic embolization of vegetation associated with aortic valve endocarditis.

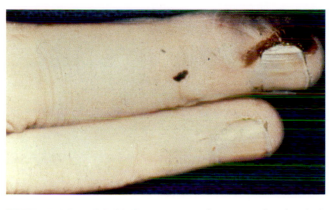

FIGURE 2.24 Digital infarct/gangrene due to peripheral emboli of aortic valve vegetations.

of Valsalva, the cerebral and carotid arteries, the branches of the abdominal aorta (the mesenteric arteries, renal artery), and more rarely limb and coronary arteries [50–60]. They occasionally rupture, causing subarachnoid or intraventricular hemorrhage or other vascular catastrophes [61–64]. Intracranial mycotic aneurysms (1.2–5% of cases) have an overall mortality of 60% but 80% if rupture should occur [62,65–67] (see Figures 2.29–2.31). Contrast-enhanced CT scanning and 3-D magnetic resonance imaging may provide adequate information but angiography remains the diagnostic imaging test of choice [65,68].

(Figures 2.37–2.40), painless red Janeway lesions on the palms and soles (Figures 2.41 a and b), and finger clubbing—which occurs late in 10–20% of patients (Figures 2.42–2.45). Mycotic aneurysms, which occur in 2–15% of patients who have IE, involve mainly the sinuses

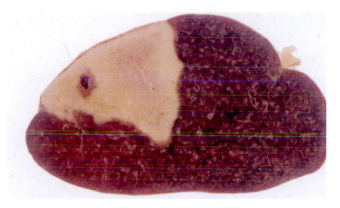

FIGURE 2.23 Large, old splenic infarct due to systemic embolus in a patient with aortic valve endocarditis. Courtesy of Dr Hani Zakhour.

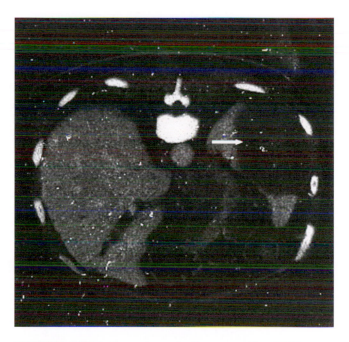

FIGURE 2.25a) Computer-assisted tomography (CAT) scan showing large splenic hemorrhagic infarct/hematoma (arrow) in a patient with prosthetic valve endocarditis on anticoagulant therapy.

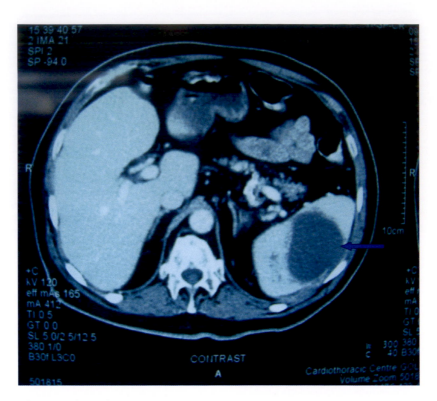

FIGURE 2.25b) CAT scan showing splenic abscess (arrow).

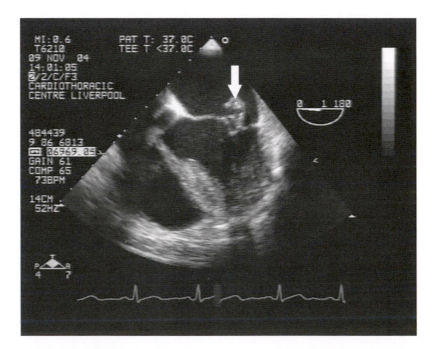

FIGURE 2.26a) Transoesophageal echocardiography shows a large vegetation on the posterior leaflet of the mitral valve (arrow) in a 53-year-old man with mitral valve prolapse, mitral regurgitation and a history of previous infective endocarditis who developed infective endocarditis due to *Staphylococcus aureus*. Fever, Janeway lesions on the right hand and left foot, left arm and facial weakness, slurred speech and mild dysphasia and a Roth spot in the left fundus were the presenting features.

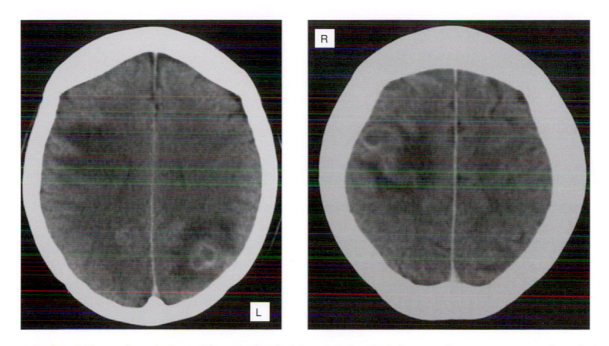

FIGURE 2.26b) A CAT scan showed a large right parietal and a left occipital cerebral abscess. Following treatment with IV flucloxacillin, cefotaxime and gentamicin for 6 weeks, the neurological deficit and the cerebral abscesses on CAT scanning resolved. He was referred electively for mitral valve replacement. Courtesy of Dr E Roberts.

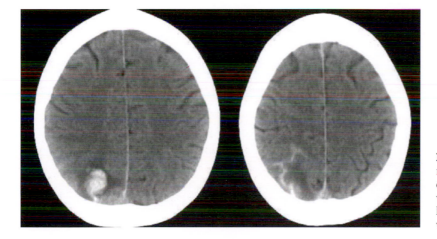

FIGURE 2.27 Two CAT scan slices showing hemorrhagic infarct in right occipital region due to systemic embolus of a vegetation from the mitral valve infected with coagulase-negative *Staphylococcus*. This patient's left homonymous hemianopia subsequently resolved with antibiotic therapy.

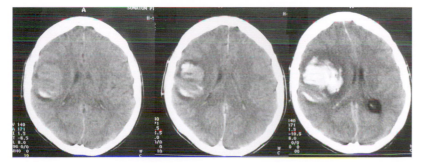

FIGURE 2.28 Three CAT scan images from a diabetic woman with a large vegetation on the mitral valve due to *Streptococcus sanguis* endocarditis. She developed a behavioral disturbance and a right hemiplegia. The left image showed an area of infarction in the left cerebral hemisphere, which progressed (central image). After rapidly lapsing into unconsciousness, a third CAT scan (right) showed severe intracerebral hemorrhage affecting the left lateral and frontal lobes and midline shift. Courtesy of Dr Chris Bellamy.

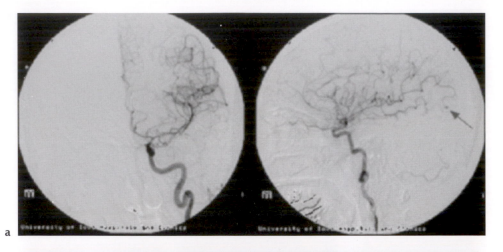

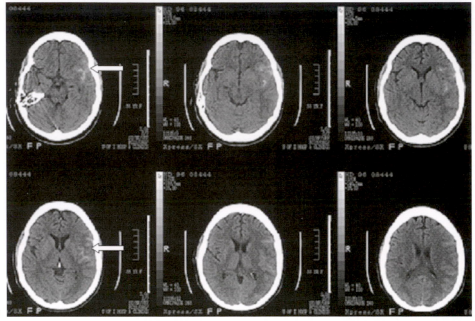

FIGURE 2.29 (a) Cerebral angiogram showing mycotic aneurysm in a distal branch of the left middle cerebral artery (arrow) in a 38-year-old male IV drug abuser with infective endocarditis presenting with severe headache. It was associated with hemorrhage in the lateral fissure (arrow) (b). Courtesy of Dr Frederick Chen. Copyright protected material used with permission of the author and the University of Iowa's Virtual Hospital, www.vh.org.

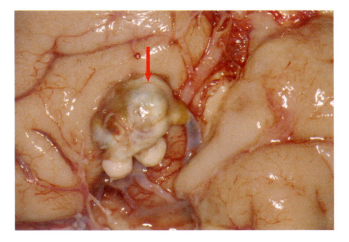

FIGURE 2.30 Mycotic aneurysms (arrow) may involve a cerebral artery in patients with infective endocarditis and result in intracerebral or subarachnoid hemorrhage. Courtesy of Dr Hani Zakhour.

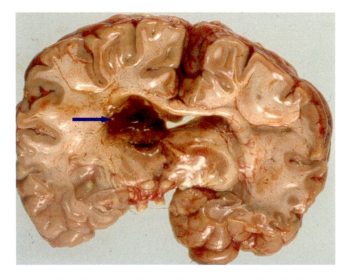

FIGURE 2.31 Ruptured mycotic aneurysms of cerebral arteries (arrow) usually cause neurological catastrophes. Courtesy of Dr Hani Zakhour.

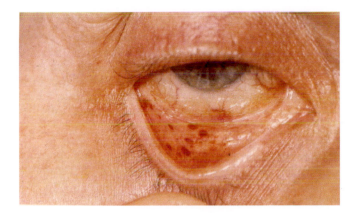

FIGURE 2.32 Subconjunctival hemorrhages.

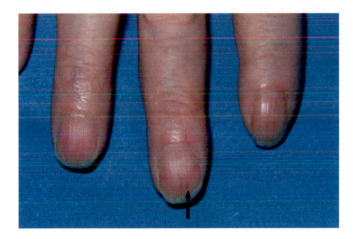

FIGURE 2.33 Splinter hemorrhage (arrow) in finger of patient with *Streptococcus faecalis* aortic valve endocarditis.

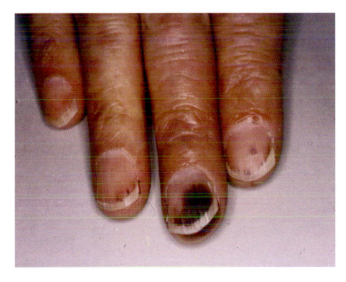

FIGURE 2.34 Extensive splinter hemorrhages in a patient with infective endocarditis of the aortic valve. Courtesy of Dr David Roberts.

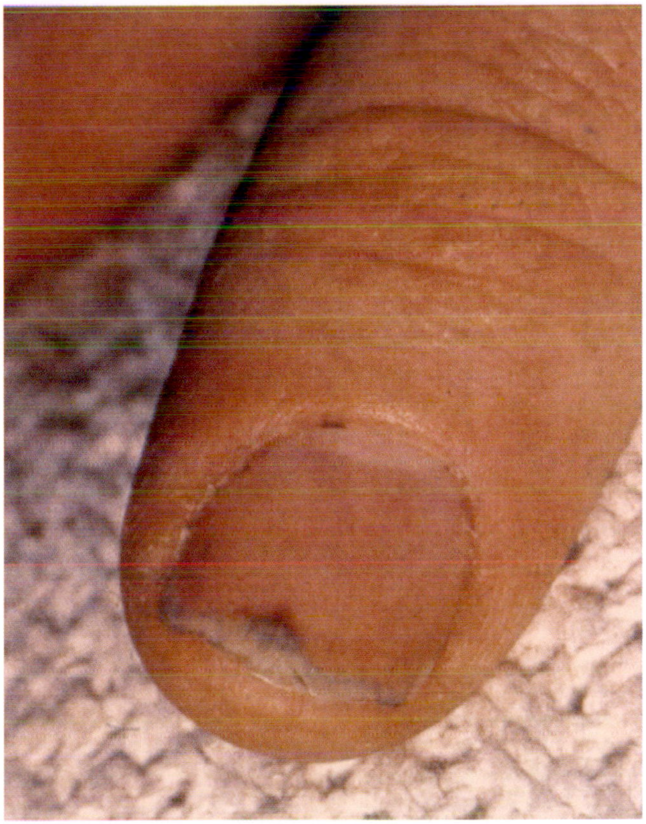

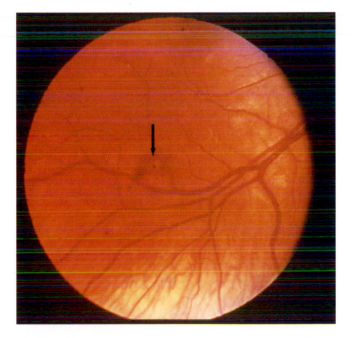

FIGURE 2.35 Splinter hemorrhage on the thumb of a patient with infective endocarditis due to viridans streptococci.

FIGURE 2.36 Roth spot (arrow) in retina of patient with infective endocarditis. Courtesy of Dr David Roberts.

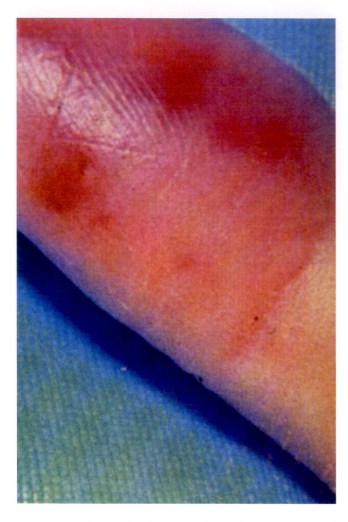

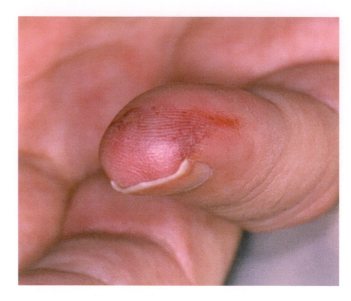

FIGURE 2.38 Osler's nodes affecting fingers of a man with infective endocarditis of the aortic valve due to *Streptococcus faecalis.*

treatment. Fifty percent of all emboli occur within 20 days and 80% within the first month after initial symptoms of IE. After an embolic complication, recurrent episodes are likely to follow, especially if vegetations persist on echocardiography. In >50% of cases, recurrence of a thromboembolic event occurs within 30 days after the first episode. It has been estimated that up to 65% of embolic events involve the central nervous system,

FIGURE 2.37 Painful, red, tender Osler's nodes on the thumb of a patient with infective endocarditis due to *Staphylococcus aureus.*

Deposits of immune complexes with complement along the renal glomerular basement membrane may cause a focal or diffuse glomerulonephritis and can be diagnosed by renal biopsy with appropriate glomeruli staining [69–71]. Arthritis and Osler's nodes have also been attributed to the local deposit of immune complexes [72–76]. Besides immune complex glomerulonephritis and septic renal infarcts, hemodynamic instability, antibiotic drug and contrast medium toxicity can be responsible for acute renal failure, which often indicates a poor prognosis.

Endopthalmitis, osteomyelitis, diskitis, and epidural abscess formation are rare complications [77–79] (Figures 2.46 a and b).

Emboli are more likely to occur with enterococci, staphylococci, Gram-negative aerobic bacilli and fungi, with large mobile vegetations and especially when the mitral valve is affected. They tend to occur early before hospital admission and within the first 2 weeks of starting

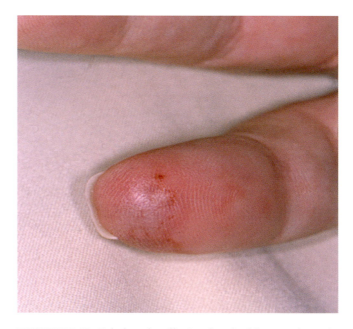

FIGURE 2.39 Osler's nodes affecting thumb of the man shown in Figure 2.38.

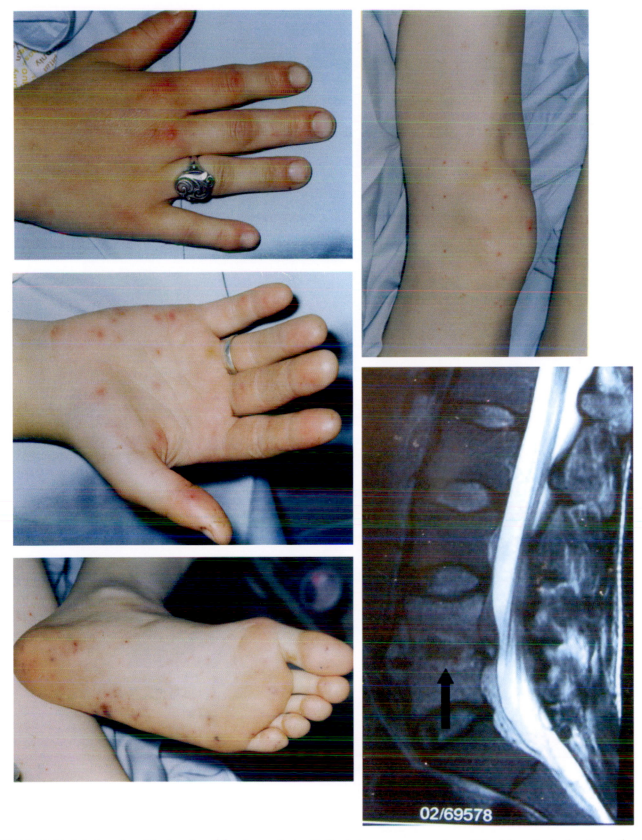

FIGURE 2.40 Osler's nodes of the hands and feet in a patient with *Staphylococcus aureus* endocarditis of the mitral valve, 8 months after presenting with acute diskitis of L4/5 (arrow).

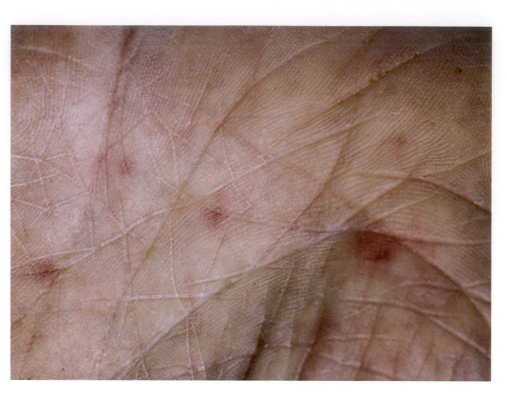

FIGURE 2.41a) Janeway macules usually seen on the palms of the hands and soles of the feet are painless, red macules. Courtesy of Dr Charlie Goldberg and Dr Josh Fierer, University of California San Diego, USA.

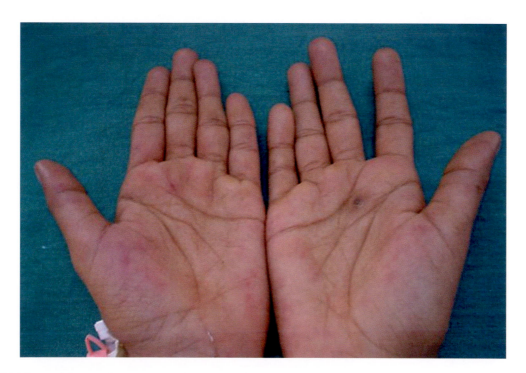

FIGURE 2.41b) These painless erythematous macules are typically distributed along the thenar and hypothenar eminences. They were due to infective endocarditis due to *Streptococcus viridans* in a woman with rheumatic mitral valve disease. Courtesy of Dr S M Divakaramenon and reproduced with permission from the BMJ Publishing Group. Heart 2005;91:516.

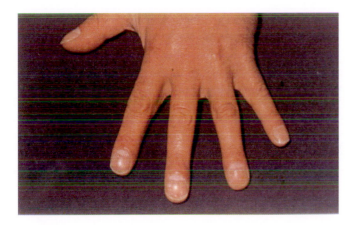

FIGURE 2.42 Finger clubbing in subacute infective endocarditis due to viridans streptococci.

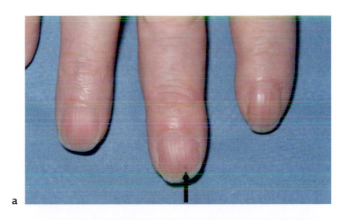

a

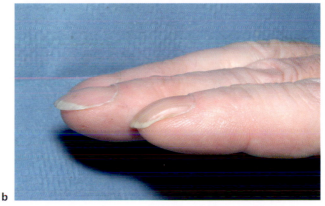

b

FIGURE 2.44 (**a** and **b**) Finger clubbing and splinter hemorrhages (arrow) in a patient with infective endocarditis of the aortic valve.

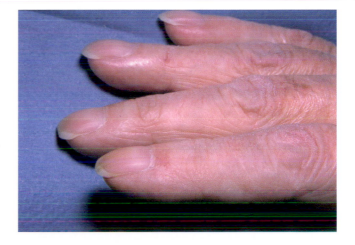

FIGURE 2.43 Finger clubbing in subacute infective endocarditis due to *Streptococcus faecalis*.

FIGURE 2.45 Finger clubbing is sometimes best appreciated by viewing the finger tips from the side.

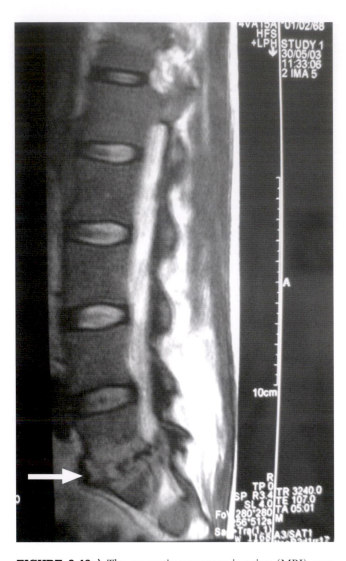

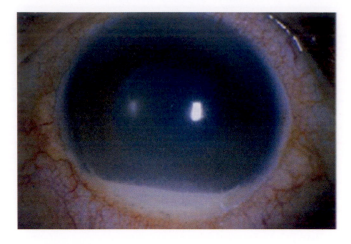

FIGURE 2.46b) Bacterial endophthalmitis causing visual loss may occur rarely as a result of streptococcal infective endocarditis (in this case *S. pneumoniae*). Courtesy of Dr S Harding.

FIGURE 2.46a) The magnetic resonance imaging (MRI) scan shows severe diskitis of L5/S1 (arrow)—an unusual result of infective endocarditis. This 34-year-old woman presented with back, suprapubic and right thigh pain, a pyrexia of 38.1°C, and a palpable tender mass over the right aspect of the sacrum. Cardiac auscultation revealed a pansystolic murmur of mitral regurgitation and blood cultures yielded *Streptococcus oralis.* Courtesy of Dr Chris Bellamy.

that the majority lodge in the middle cerebral artery territory, and that the associated mortality is high [80].

SPECIFIC MANIFESTATIONS

Right-sided Endocarditis
In patients with right-sided IE, the tricuspid valve is most frequently involved (80%) (Figure 2.47), pulmonary infarcts are often followed by lung abscesses, and pleural effusions occur [81–84] (Figure 2.48). Hemoptysis can be fatal [64]. Mycotic aneurysms of the pulmonary arteries

may also be complicated by potentially fatal pulmonary hemorrhage. Peripheral emboli and immunological vascular phenomena generally do not occur but massive pulmonary embolism of large vegetations can be fatal (Figure 2.49). The main cause is intravenous drug abuse but others include pacemaker infection, central IV lines, skin and gynecological infections, and bacteremia in patients who have congenital cardiac lesions [85,86]. In IV drug abuse, the prognosis of right-sided IE is favorable (4–5% mortality) but recurrences are frequent (30%) [87,88]. When endocarditis is associated with infection of pacemakers (Figures 2.50a–d), automatic implantable defibrillators, central IV or Hickman lines or other foreign bodies, e.g. septal occluder devices, tube grafts etc., the objects need to be removed in order to maximize the chance of successful treatment and antimicrobial therapy is required for 4–6 weeks [89] (Figures 2.51 and 2.52). *S. aureus* and *S. epidermidis* are responsible for 50% and 25% of pacemaker infections respectively. Special techniques have been reported for removal of infected material associated with large vegetations [90,91], but not infrequently open heart surgery is the only option (Figures 2.53 and 2.54). Forceful traction on retained electrodes is hazardous, especially on actively fixed, screw-in atrial leads, when myocardium may be removed and myocardial perforation and cardiac tamponade may occur (Figure 2.55).

Prosthetic Valve Endocarditis
When prosthetic valves are affected (accounts for 5–15% of all cases in developed countries [92,93]), abscesses are particularly frequent, extending beyond the prosthetic ring into the annulus and periannular tissue (Figure 2.56). Conduction system disturbance and even purulent pericarditis

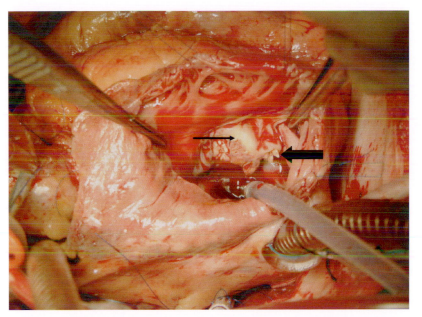

FIGURE 2.47 Tricuspid valve endocarditis following diagnostic cardiac catheterization is exceedingly rare but in this case was due to *Staphylococcus aureus*. A valvular abscess (thin arrow) and vegetation (thick arrow) on the tricuspid valve are shown. Courtesy of Mr Walid Dihmis.

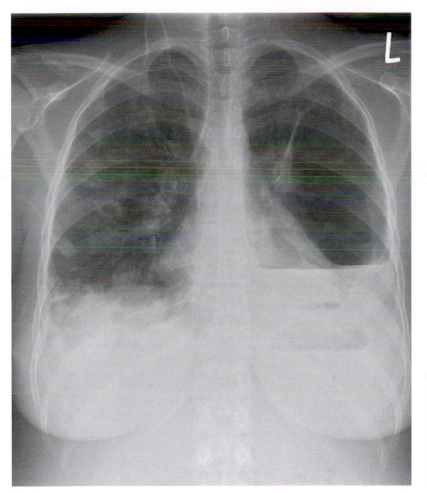

FIGURE 2.48 Chest X-ray showing many of the features typical of right-sided infective endocarditis complicated by septic pulmonary emboli. Multiple alveolar opacities are noted in the right lung. Abscess formation in the left lung has caused a bronchopleural fistula, pneumothorax, and empyema, hence the fluid level. Courtesy of Dr Brad Munt and Dr Rob Moss. Heart 2003;89:577–581. Reproduced with permission from the BMJ Publishing Group.

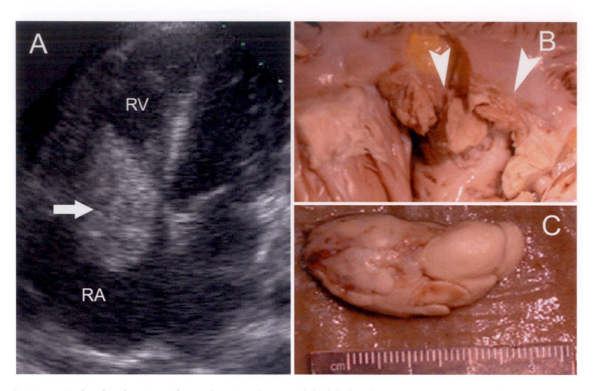

FIGURE 2.49 A. Apical 4-chamber view of TTE showing a large, mobile, lobulated vegetation (arrow) partially obstructing the tricuspid valve and prolapsing into the right ventricle (RV). Tricuspid valve endocarditis was due to *Streptococcus agalactiae*. RA = right atrium. B. The tricuspid valve is eroded and associated with a myocardial abscess (arrowheads). C. Death was due to massive pulmonary embolism. Autopsy revealed complete obstruction of the right pulmonary artery by this 3 × 2 cm mass, representing a fragment of the bacterial vegetation. *S. agalactiae* lack fibrinolysin production, which might explain the unusual, large, friable vegetations and their frequent embolisation. Courtesy of Dr. C B Marcu and reproduced with permission from the BMJ Publishing Group. Heart 2005;91:279.

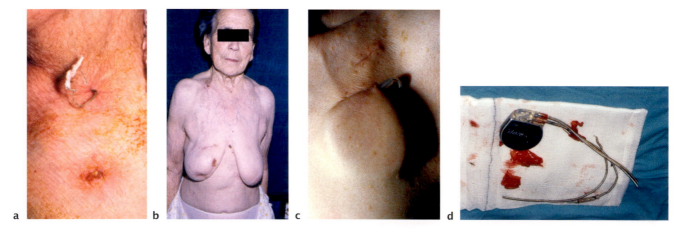

FIGURE 2.50 (a–d) Eroded pacemakers can become infected and should be removed. Pacemaker pocket infection with *Staphylococcus aureus* may result in infective endocarditis with vegetations on the endocardial lead and tricuspid valve. **d)** Explanted infected dual chamber pacemaker and leads.

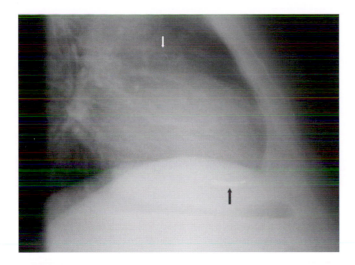

FIGURE 2.51 This patient with an infected automatic implantable defibrillator (AICD) and staphylococcal septicemia had the device explanted. However, the ventricular lead could not be removed either by manual traction or using the excimer lead removal system. The fractured stretched electrode embolized into the pulmonary artery (white arrow) and the tined electrode tip remained firmly anchored in the right ventricular apex (black arrow).

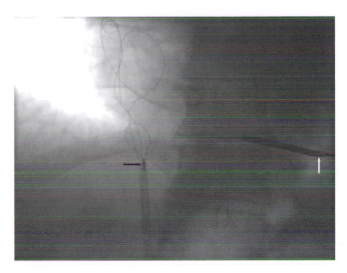

FIGURE 2.52 With infected pacing systems such as this, every effort must be made to remove all hardware—to avoid subsequent septicemia and endocarditis. A Dotter retrieval catheter (black arrow) was used to capture the loops of bare electrode in the pulmonary artery, and withdraw them into the right atrium and down the inferior vena cava. However, despite strong tension the electrode tip remained firmly adherent to the right ventricular apex (white arrow).

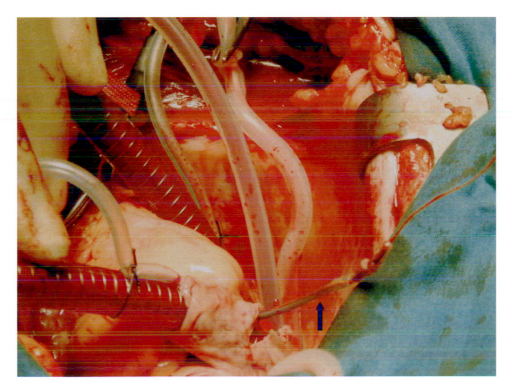

FIGURE 2.53 This patient underwent a thoracotomy and atriotomy on cardiopulmonary bypass in order to remove the infected electrode (arrow). Even then the lead could not be freed by simple traction, and dissection away from the ventricular muscle was necessary.

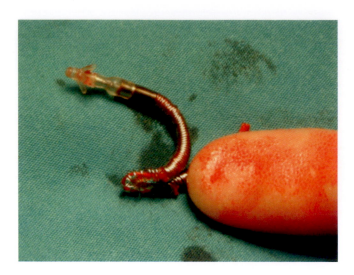

FIGURE 2.54 Tip of tined ventricular AICD lead removed surgically from the right ventricular apex.

are serious complications. The diagnosis requires a high index of suspicion from the clinician [94]. Ring or septal abscess, fistulous tract, and dehiscence of the prosthesis are frequent autopsy findings. Vegetations can interfere with disk function, causing obstruction and/or regurgitation. In bioprosthetic valve IE, the anatomic lesions vary between limited leaflet infection and disseminated infection and valve destruction [95] (Figure 2.57).

Early The microbiology of early (<60 days) PVE (which still accounts for 0.4–1.2% of cases) and of those occurring

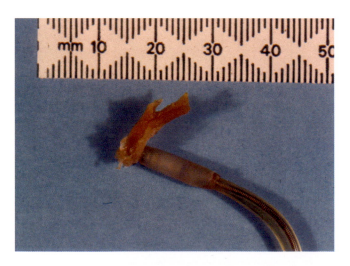

FIGURE 2.55 Removing infected permanent pacemaker electrodes, especially actively fixed leads, may be impossible by direct traction. Persistence may result in removal of myocardium, cardiac perforation, cardiac tamponade, and death; this may be more of a problem in the thinner atrium. Excimer laser lead-extraction may be possible but open heart surgery may be necessary, especially if the electrode is adherent to the tricuspid valve leaflet as well.

within the first year of surgery is distinctive [96,97]. *S. aureus* and *S. epidermidis* predominate (45–50%), followed by Gram-negative aerobic bacilli and fungi. Streptococci and enterococci are less common, accounting for <10% of cases. Contamination occurs intraoperatively via the wound or from the extracorporeal circulation or postoperatively from IV catheters, arterial lines, urethral catheters, and endotracheal tubes. Of the staphylococci, coagulase-negative staphylococci predominate, particularly *S. epidermidis*—an increasing number of which are methicillin-resistant. *S. aureus* PVE has a high mortality and surgery should be considered early [98].

Late In late (>60 days) PVE, the bacteriology more closely resembles that of community-acquired native IE [44,99] although staphylococci are still important causative organisms (Figure 2.58). The risk of IE after cardiac surgical and interventional procedures has been discussed by de Gevigney et al [100]. The incidence may be higher in tissue than in mechanical valves [101] (Figure 2.59).

Fungal Endocarditis

Fungal endocarditis is frequently characterized by negative blood cultures and a paucity of physical signs [102–107]. The majority of fungal endocarditis is caused by candida or aspergillus infection. Fever, changing murmurs, and the presence of peripheral emboli—commonly of large vessels, in the brain, gut, kidneys, coronary arteries, and the limbs—are the most common signs of fungal endocarditis. Although blood cultures are generally negative in fungal endocarditis, 83–95% are positive in those with candida infection (Figures 2.60 and 2.61). Culture of a peripheral arterial embolus may provide the best and only clue to the presence of fungal endocarditis and the specimen can be examined microscopically for hyphae (Figure 2.62). Routine serology has been useful in deep-seated cryptococcosis and histoplasmosis and although candida precipitins and aspergillus antigens and antibodies might provide supportive diagnostic evidence of fungal infection, their sensitivity and specificity are disappointing [108–111]. Fungal vegetations are frequently large (10–30 mm diameter), bulky and friable, and valvular or endocardial in position [112]. Echocardiography and transesophageal echocardiography (TEE) in particular are most important in establishing an etiological diagnosis, for defining the anatomical extent of the valvular disease and for guiding the surgical strategy [113]. Emboli are frequently large and multiple, cause considerable functional and neurological damage, and lead to the associated high mortality [107]. Metastatic abscesses are another frequent complication—the heart and kidneys being involved most commonly [114,115] (Figures 2.63–2.65). Special

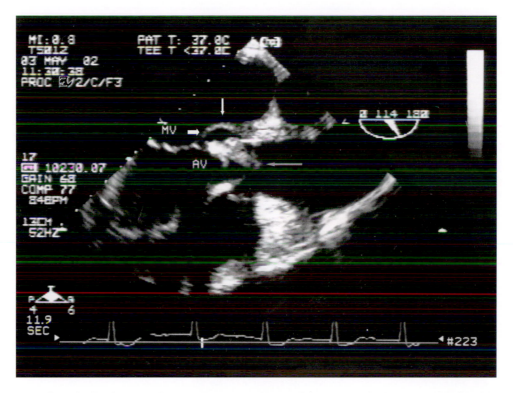

FIGURE 2.56 Transesophageal echo showing a large vegetation on a bioprosthetic aortic valve (gray arrow) infected by coagulase-negative *Staphylococcus*. A large paravalvular abscess is clearly visible (twin white arrows).

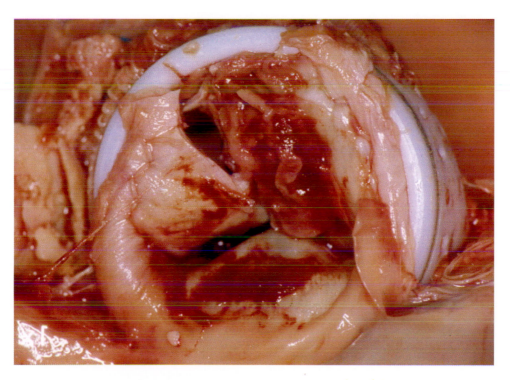

FIGURE 2.57 Infected aortic valve bioprosthesis destroyed by *Staphylococcus aureus* endocarditis.

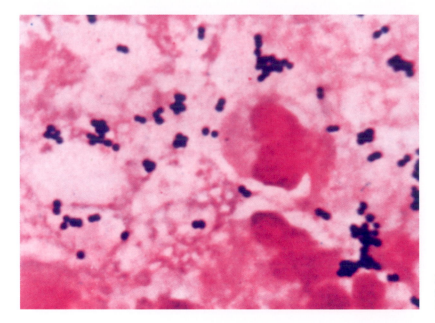

FIGURE 2.58 Gram-positive *Staphylococcus aureus* seen by histological examination of infected tissue adherent to an infected prosthetic valve.

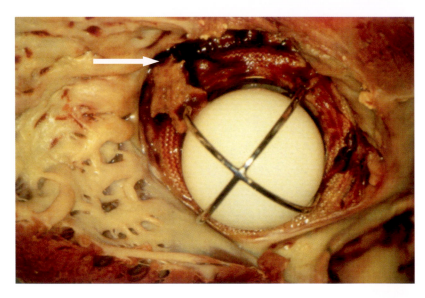

FIGURE 2.59 Infected Starr–Edwards mechanical prosthesis as a result of *Staphylococcus epidermidis* infection (arrow).

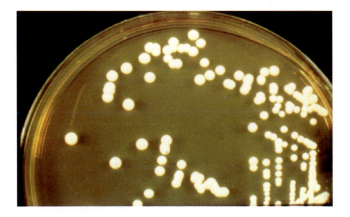

FIGURE 2.60a) Colonies of *Candida albicans* growing on Sabouraud's medium.

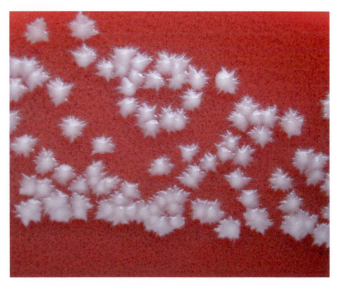

FIGURE 2.60b) Opaque colonies of *Candida albicans* growing on blood agar. Courtesy of Dr. John Cunniffe.

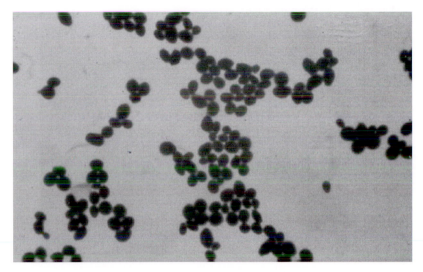

FIGURE 2.61 Yeasts visualized microscopically.

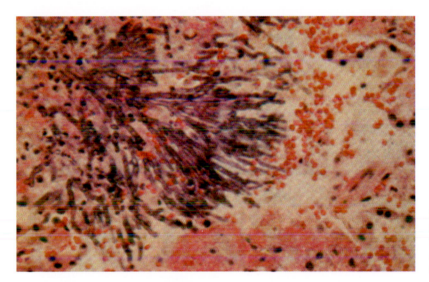

FIGURE 2.62 Culture of a peripheral arterial embolus or histological examination may provide the best and only evidence of fungal endocarditis. This specimen shows fungal hyphae due to *Aspergillus* infection of the tricuspid valve of an IV drug abuser.

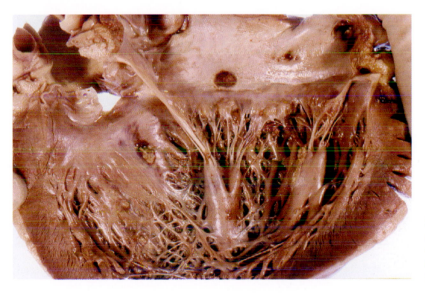

FIGURE 2.63 Myocardial abscess due to *Candida albicans* infective endocarditis. The valve and the endocardial surface bear well-defined red-gray vegetations in this 46-year-old woman dying of acute lymphoblastic leukemia. Courtesy of Dr John Gosney.

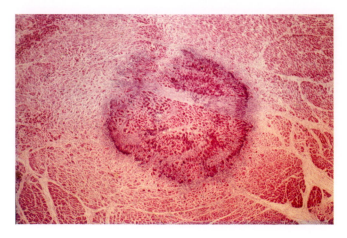

FIGURE 2.64 Histology of myocardial abscess due to *Candida* infection, showing a large aggregate of fungal hyphae within the myocardium. The specimen is stained with the periodic acid–Schiff (PAS) method, which brings up the carbohydrate in the fungal hyphae allowing them to be seen easily. Courtesy of Dr John Gosney.

stains can help to identify fungal hyphae histologically (Figure 2.66).

Medical treatment combined with early surgery is the mainstay of treatment. Surgery (valve replacement) should be performed as soon as the bulky vegetations are diagnosed in order to prevent the high rate (68%) of embolization. Fungal endocarditis may complicate prolonged antibiotic treatment of PVE and prophylactic oral nystatin may be valuable [116].

Blood Culture-negative Endocarditis

Blood culture-negative endocarditis (CNE) (5–10%) is usually due to patients having been treated with antibiotics

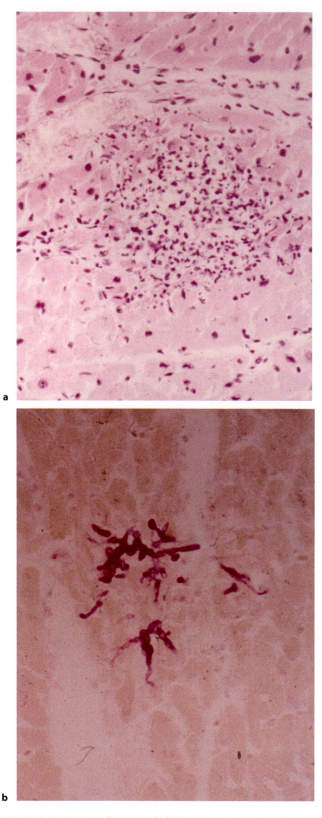

FIGURE 2.66 Fungal myocardial abscess stained with hematoxylin and eosin (H&E) appears as an acute inflammatory focus (a) but fungal hyphae can be seen clearly when stained by the PAS method (b).

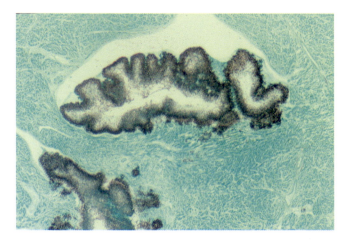

FIGURE 2.65 Histology of myocardial abscess due to *Candida* infection stained with the Grocott silver impregnation method. Here, the silver is precipitated from a silver salt onto the hyphae and looks black under the microscope. The counterstain is called "light green". Courtesy of Dr John Gosney.

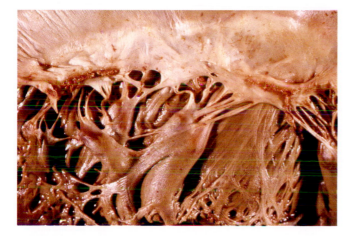

FIGURE 2.67 Marantic vegetations as seen on this mitral valve are sometimes associated with malignant and/or emaciating illness. The vegetations tend to be small. These were an incidental finding in an 80-year-old woman dying of carcinoma of the pancreas.

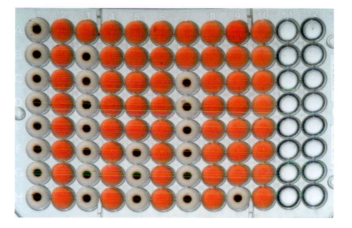

FIGURE 2.68 *Brucella* microagglutination test. This test is used to determine the relative concentration of *Brucella* antibodies (both IgG and IgM) present in the patient's serum. The serum is incubated with a saffranin-stained *Brucella abortus* antigen. The positive reaction is detected by an absence of pellet formation due to the formation of antigen–antibody complexes. Courtesy of Dr Mike Rothburn.

prior to the blood cultures being taken. Other causes include fungal infections, fastidious slow-growing organisms, e.g. *Brucella* spp., *Mycoplasma* spp., *Bartonella* spp., *Chlamydia* spp., *Histoplasma* spp., *Legionella* spp., and *Coxiella burnetii*, and "noninfective" endocarditis as seen in systemic lupus erythematosus and in terminal malignant disease (so-called "marantic endocarditis") [117–128] (Figure 2.67; Table 2.1). However, systemic lupus erythematosus and IE can coexist [129].

Some of the more unusual infections have certain clinical features that are suggestive. For example, Q-fever endocarditis often occurs in patients in contact with farm animals, frequently involving the aortic valve but also the mitral and prosthetic valves. Liver involvement, thrombocytopenia, and purpura are common [130,131]. Vegetations are usually small. *Brucella* endocarditis is also found in patients in contact with cattle and goats, usually farmers and veterinary surgeons. Again the aortic valve is more frequently affected and aneurysms of the sinus of

Valsalva with intramyocardial spread are common. PVE has been reported [132].

Advances in serology, histology, and molecular biology have helped in establishing the diagnosis in CNE. Serological tests (antibodies, precipitins) may be helpful in these situations, particularly for rickettsia such as *Coxiella*, *Brucella*, or *Chlamydia* [133] (Figures 2.68–2.70;

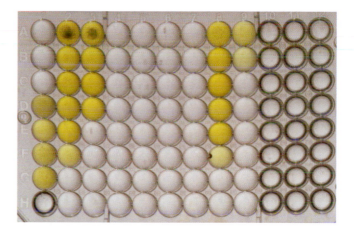

FIGURE 2.69 *Brucella* enzyme immunoassay. This test is in two stages. In the first stage "U"-bottomed microtiter plates are coated with *Brucella abortus* antigen suspension. In the second stage, the patient's serum is added. If antibodies are present, these form a complex with the antigens and are fixed. The complex is detected by adding an enzyme-labeled monoclonal antibody. When substrate is added, a positive reaction is indicated by yellow coloration. This detects both IgG and IgM antibodies. 1–12 = different patients; A–H = serum samples, serially double diluted from one well to the next until the antibody (if present) is too dilute to be detected. The final dilution is expressed as a "titer". Courtesy of Dr Mike Rothburn.

TABLE 2.1 Causes of Culture-Negative Endocarditis

Previous antibiotics
Fastidious organisms
  Nutritionally dependent streptococci
  The HACEK group of oropharyngeal flora
  Bacterial L-forms and anaerobes
  Brucella, Neisseria, Legionella
  Nocardia, mycobacteria
  Mycoplasma pneumoniae
Cell-dependent organisms
  Chlamydia, Coxiella, Bartonella
Fungi
Major immune activation—"Endocarditis lente"

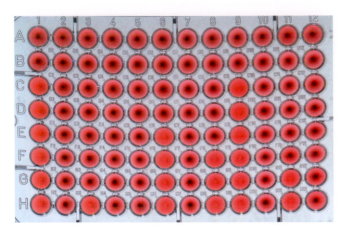

FIGURE 2.70 Complement fixation test (CFT). This is a two-stage test for the presence of antibody in serum (both IgG and IgM). In *stage 1*, the serum and known antigen react together in the presence of added complement. If antigen combines with antibody, the complement is fixed. This fixation is detected in *stage 2* by the addition of sensitized sheep red blood cells (coated with antibody). The picture shows positives as buttons of settled red blood cells. Negatives show uniform lysis caused by free (unfixed) complement. This test is used for detection of various bacteria which may cause culture-negative infective endocarditis notably, *Brucella*, *Coxiella* (Q-fever), and *Chlamydia psittaci*. Courtesy of Dr Mike Rothburn.

Table 2.2). Although *Coxiella* (a strict intracellular Gram-negative organism) may be found by Giemsa staining of the excised valve, endocarditis is best diagnosed by IgG (>1/800) and IgA (>1/100) titers to phase I antigen using the microimmunofluorescence (MIF) test [133–137]. For *Brucella* spp. (a facultative intracellular Gram-negative bacillus), high titers of specific IgG and IgM antibodies by microagglutination, enzyme immunoassay, or complement fixation techniques are diagnostic (see

TABLE 2.2 Serologic Tests Used in the Diagnosis of Infective Endocarditis [149]

Microorganism	Serologic technique	Cut-off value
Coxiella burnetii	Indirect immunofluorescence	IgG to phase 1 >1:800
Bartonella species	Indirect immunofluorescence	IgG >1:1600
Chlamydia species	Indirect immunofluorescence	IgG >1:128
Legionella pneumophila	Indirect immunofluorescence	IgG >1:128
Mycoplasma pneumoniae	IgM enzyme immunoassay	Optical density >control
	Complement fixation	>1:64
Brucella melitensis	Wright's serum agglutination test	IgG >1:80
	Card test	Qualitative test: positive or negative

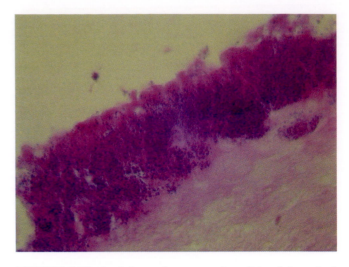

FIGURE 2.71 *Staphylococcal aureus* endocarditis of the mitral valve. Darkly staining Gram-positive cocci in a vegetation revealed by the Brown–Brenn tissue Gram stain. Original magnification ×400. Courtesy of Drs H. Lepidi and D. Raoult.

Figures 2.68–2.70). Special histological stains (Figures 2.71 and 2.72; Table 2.3), immunohistology (Figures 2.73 and 2.74; Table 2.4), and occasionally electron microscopy can help visualize organisms in valvular and other tissues

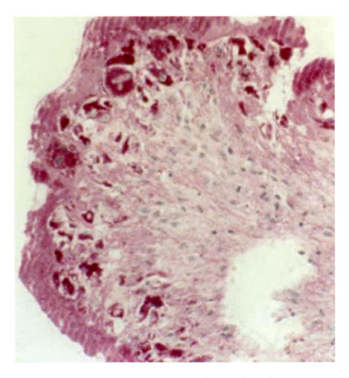

FIGURE 2.72 *Tropheryma whipplei* endocarditis. Foamy macrophages containing the characteristic inclusion bodies in an aortic valve from a patient with Whipple endocarditis. Periodic acid–Schiff stain. Original magnification ×250. Courtesy of Drs H. Lepidi and D. Raoult.

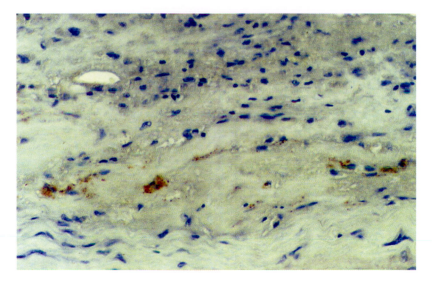

FIGURE 2.73 Q-fever endocarditis. Immunohistochemical detection of *Coxiella burnetii* in a resected aortic valve from a patient with Q-fever endocarditis, using a monoclonal antibody and hematoxylin counterstain. This immunoperoxidase stain demonstrates the intracytoplasmic, small coccobacillus *Coxiella burnetii*. The inclusion bodies appear an orange-brown color. Original magnification ×400. Courtesy of Drs H. Lepidi and D. Raoult.

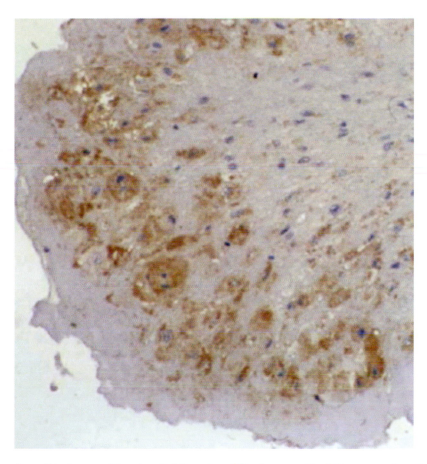

FIGURE 2.74 Whipple endocarditis: Immunohistochemical detection of *Tropheryma whipplei* in a resected aortic valve from a patient with Whipple endocarditis, using a polyclonal antibody and hematoxylin counterstain—immunoperoxidase method. Bacilli are packed as coarse granular immunopositive material in foamy macrophage cytoplasm. Original magnification ×250. Courtesy of Drs H. Lepidi and D. Raoult.

TABLE 2.3 Histological Stains of Use in the Diagnosis of Infective Endocarditis [149]

Tissue stain	Detected microorganisms
Giemsa	Any bacterium
Tissue Gram	
– Brown–Brenn	Gram-positive bacteria
– Brown–Hopps	Gram-negative bacteria
Periodic acid–Schiff	*Tropheryma whipplei*, fungi
Warthin–Starry	*Bartonella* species
Ziehl–Neelsen	Acid-fast bacilli
Gimenez	*Coxiella burnetii*, *Legionella* species
Grocott–Gomori methenamine silver	Fungi

TABLE 2.4 Immunohistological techniques

Immunoperoxidase stain
Enzyme-linked immunosorbent assay (ELISA)
Enzyme-linked immunofluorescent assay (ELIFA)
Direct immunofluorescence using fluorescein-conjugated monoclonal antibodies

removed surgically [138–143]. Bacterial polymerase chain reaction (PCR) analysis for the amplification of bacterial DNA can be crucial in confirming the diagnosis in CNE, e.g. *Tropheryma whipplei* or *Bartonella* spp., and such molecular analysis has been recently implemented into the

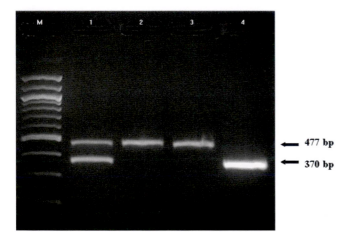

FIGURE 2.75 Polymerase chain reaction (PCR) products visualized by ethidium bromide staining on a 2% agarose gel undergoing electrophoresis. PCR product of 370 bp indicates a presence of bacterial DNA in the sample. The band of 477 bp corresponds to an internal standard. PCR fragment from lane 4 was cut, DNA purified by Gel Extraction Kit and directly sequenced using BidDye Terminator kit on ABI3100-Avant sequencer (Applied Biosystems). The sequence was compared with sequences obtained from public domain databases (NCBI) for determination of pathogen identity. In this case *Actinobacillus actinomycetemcomitans* was identified as the cause of culture-negative infective endocarditis. Courtesy of Tomas Freiberger, Center for Cardiovascular Surgery and Transplantation-CKTCH, Brno, Czech Republic.

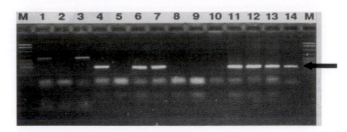

FIGURE 2.76 Polymerase chain reaction (PCR) and DNA amplification techniques can detect DNA from microorganisms that are present in too few numbers to be visualized or when growth characteristics are such that there would be a delay in diagnosis. Advantages of the technique are speed, automation, high degree of specificity and sensitivity, crude extract is satisfactory, and the inoculum need not be viable. The amplified DNA products can then be visualized by agarose gel electrophoresis and staining of DNA with ethidium bromide, which intercalates between the nucleotide bases and fluoresces under ultraviolet light. Here fragments of the expected size (bp) of DNA from *T. whipplei* are identified (arrow) by agarose gel electrophoresis. This organism may cause severe spondylodiskitis and infective endocarditis. Courtesy of Professor M. Altwegg, Department of Microbiology, University of Zurich, Switzerland.

newest revision of the Duke criteria [144–148] (Figures 2.75 and 2.76). The main advantages of the methods are that they can be used on most types of clinical material, including valvular specimens, are culture-independent and that through the incorporation of "broad-spectrum" primers, almost any bacteria can be detected in a single reaction. Identification of the microorganism from which amplified DNA is derived can be easily achieved by determining the nucleotide base sequence of a PCR product and then comparing it with reference sequences in databases such as Genbank or the European Molecular Biology Laboratory database.

These additional tests may not only improve the sensitivity of the diagnosis, but may also improve the outcome by increasing the specificity of the antibiotic treatment.

REFERENCES

1. Bayer AS, Bolger AF, Taubert KA, et al. Diagnosis and management of infective endocarditis and its complications. Circulation 1998;98:2936–2948.
2. Chambers HF, Korzeniowski OM, Sande MA. *Staphylococcus aureus* endocarditis: clinical manifestations in addicts and non-addicts. Medicine 1983;62:170–177.
3. Espersen F, Frimodt-Moller N. *Staphylococcus aureus* endocarditis. A review of 119 cases. Arch Intern Med 1986;146:1118–1121.
4. Terpenning MS, Buggy BP, Kauffman CA. Infective endocarditis: clinical features in young and elderly patients. Am J Med 1987;83:626–634.

5. Durack DT. Infective and non-infective endocarditis. In: Hurst JW, ed. The Heart, Arteries and Veins, 7th edn. New York: McGraw-Hill; 1990:1230–1255.

6. Ferrieri P, Gewitz MH, Gerber MA, et al. Unique features of infective endocarditis in childhood. AHA Scientific Statement. Circulation 2002;105:2115–2127.

7. Varma MP, McCluskey DR, Khan MM, et al. Heart failure associated with infective endocarditis. A review of 40 cases. Br Heart J 1986;55:191–197.

8. Mills J, Utley J, Abbott J. Heart failure in infective endocarditis: predisposing factors, course and treatment. Chest 1974;66:151–157.

9. Smith RH, Radford DJ, Clark RA, Julian DG. Infectious endocarditis: a survey of cases in the South East region of Scotland between 1969 and 1972. Thorax 1976;31:373–379.

10. Lerner PI, Weinstein L. Infective endocarditis in the antibiotic era. N Engl J Med 1966;274:199–206; 259–66; 388–393.

11. Weinstein L. Life-threatening complications of infective endocarditis and their management. Arch Intern Med 1986;146:953–957.

12. Lam D, Emilson B, Rapaport E. Four-valve endocarditis with associated right ventricular mural vegetations. Am Heart J 1988;115:189–192.

13. James PR, Dawson D, Hardman SM. Eustachian valve endocarditis diagnosed by transoesophageal echocardiography. Heart 1999;81:91.

14. Palakodeti V, Keen WD Jr, Rickman LS, Blanchard DG. Eustachian valve endocarditis: detection with multiplanar transesophageal echocardiography. Clin Cardiol 1997;20:579–580.

15. San Roman JA, Vilacosta I, Sarria C, et al. Eustachian valve endocarditis: is it worth searching for? Am Heart J 2001;142:1037–1040.

16. Sawhney N, Palakodeti V, Raisinghani A, et al. Eustachian valve endocarditis: a case series and analysis of the literature. J Am Soc Echocardiogr 2001;14:1139–1142.

17. Thomas D, Desruennes M, Jault F, Isnard R, Gandjbakhch I. Cardiac and extracardiac abscesses in infective endocarditis. Arch Mal Coeur 1993;86(Suppl 12):1825–1837.

18. Arnett EN, Roberts WC. Valve ring abscess in active endocarditis. Frequency, location and clues to clinical diagnosis from the study of 95 necropsy patients. Circulation 1976;54:140–145.

19. Sandler MA, Kotler MN, Bloom RD, Jacobson L. Pericardial abscess extending from mitral vegetation: an unusual complication of infective endocarditis. Am Heart J 1989;118:857–859.

20. Oakley CM. Perivalvular abscesses in infective endocarditis. Eur Heart J 1999;20:170–171.

21. Hwang SW, Yucel EK, Bernard S. Aortic root abscess with fistula formation. Chest 1997;111:1436–1438.

22. Piper C, Hetzer R, Korfer F, et al. The importance of secondary mitral valve involvement in primary aortic valve endocarditis: The mitral kissing vegetation. Eur Heart J 2002;23:79–86.

23. Vaghjimal A, Lutwick LI, Chapnick EK, Greengart A. Interventricular septal endocarditis. South Med J 1998;91:43–44.

24. Behnam R. Aortico-left atrial fistula in aortic valve endocarditis. Chest 1992;102:1271–1273.

25. Anguera I, Quaglio G, Miro JM, et al. Aortocardiac fistulas complicating infective endocarditis. Am J Cardiol 2001;87:652–654.

26. Bussani R, Sinagra G, Poletti A, et al. Cardiac tamponade: an unusual, fatal complication of infective endocarditis. G Ital Cardiol 1999;29:1512–1516.

27. DiNubile MJ, Calderwood SB, Steinhaus DM, Karchmer AW. Cardiac conduction abnormalities complicating native valve active infective endocarditis. Am J Cardiol 1986;58:1213–1217.

28. Brogdon BG. Sinus of Valsalva aneurysm secondary to aortic valve endocarditis. Invest Radiol 1988;23:222–223.

29. Charney R, Keltz TN, Attai L, et al. Acute valvular obstruction from streptococcal endocarditis. Am Heart J 1993;125:544–547.

30. Bhagwat AR, Patil RB, Loya YS, Sharma S. Subaortic aneurysm in infective endocarditis. Am Heart J 1991;122:588–589.

31. McDonald CL, Crafton EM, Covin FA, et al. Pericarditis: a probable complication of endocarditis due to *Haemophilus influenzae.* Clin Infect Dis 1994;18:648–649.

32. Wilson WR, Giuliani ER, Danielson GK, Geraci JE. Management of complications of infective endocarditis. Mayo Clinic Proc 1982;57:162–170.

33. Perera R, Noack S, Dong W. Acute myocardial infarction due to septic coronary embolism. N Engl J Med 2000;342:977–978.

34. Jeremias A, Casserly I, Estess JM, et al. Acute myocardial infarction after aortic valve endocarditis. Am J Med 2001;110:417–418.

35. Anguera I, Quaglio G, Ferrer B, et al. Sudden death in *Staphylococcus aureus*-associated infective endocarditis due to perforation of a free-wall myocardial abscess. Scand J Infect Dis 2001;33:622–625.

36. Chikwe J, Barnard J, Pepper JR. Myocardial abscess. Images in cardiology. Heart 2004;90:597.

37. Shackcloth MJ, Dihmis WC. Contained rupture of a myocardial abscess in the free wall of the left ventricle. Ann Thorac Surg 2001;72:617–619.

38. Ting W, Silverman NA, Arzouman DA, Levitsky S. Splenic septic emboli in endocarditis. Circulation 1990;82(Suppl IV):105–109.

39. Millaire A, Leroy O, Gaday V, et al. Incidence and prognosis of embolic events and metastatic infections in infective endocarditis. Eur Heart J 1997;18:677–684.

40. Weinstein L, Rubin RH. Infective endocarditis—1973. Prog Cardiovasc Dis 1973;16:239–274.

41. Lutwick LI, Gradon JD, Chapnick EK, et al. *Haemophilus parainfluenzae* endocarditis treated with vegetectomy and complicated by late, fatal splenic rupture. Pediatr Infect Dis J 1991;10:778–781.

42. Pringle SD, McCartney AC, Cobbe SM. Spontaneous splenic rupture as complication of infective endocarditis. Int J Cardiol 1988;19:384–386.

43. Heiro M, Nikoskelainen J, Engblom E, et al. Neurological manifestations of infective endocarditis: a 17-year experience in a teaching hospital in Finland. Arch Intern Med 2000;160:2781–2787.

44. Mylonakis E, Calderwood SB. Infective endocarditis in adults. N Engl J Med 2001;345:1318–1330.

45. Salgado AV, Furlan AJ, Keys TF, et al. Neurologic complications of endocarditis: a 12 year experience. Neurology 1989;39:173–178.

46. Delahaye JP, Poncet P, Malquarti V, et al. Cerebrovascular accidents in infective endocarditis: role of anticoagulation. Eur Heart J 1990;11:1074–1078.

47. Weeks SG, Silva C, Auer RN, et al. Encephalopathy with staphylococcal endocarditis: multiple neuropathological findings. Can J Neurol Sci 2001;28:260–264.

48. Cabell CH, Pond KK, Peterson GE, et al. The risk of stroke and death in patients with aortic and mitral valve endocarditis. Am Heart J 2001;142:75–80.

49. Kelly J, Barnass S. *Staphylococcus aureus* endocarditis presenting as meningitis and mimicking meningococcal sepsis. Int J Clin Pract 1999;53:306–307.

50. Hubautt JJ, Albat B, Frapier JM, Chaptal PA. Mycotic aneurysm of the extracranial carotid artery: an uncommon complication of bacterial endocarditis. Ann Vasc Surg 1997;11:634–636.

51. Silver SG. Ruptured mycotic aneurysm of the superior mesenteric artery that was due to *Cardiobacterium endocarditis*. Clin Infect Dis 1999;29:1573–1574.

52. Ohebshalom MM, Tash JA, Coll D, et al. Massive hematuria due to right renal artery mycotic pseudoaneurysm in a patient with subacute bacterial endocarditis. Urology 2001;58:607.

53. Cakalagaoglu C, Keser N, Alhan C. Brucella-mediated prosthetic valve endocarditis with brachial artery mycotic aneurysm. J Heart Valve Dis 1999;8:586–590.

54. McKee MA, Ballard JC. Mycotic aneurysm of the tibio-peroneal arteries. Ann Vasc Surg 1999;13:188–190.

55. Mann CF, Barker SG. Occluded mycotic popliteal aneurysm secondary to infective endocarditis. Eur J Vasc Endovasc Surg 1999;18:169–170.

56. Safar HA, Cina CS. Ruptured mycotic aneurysm of the popliteal artery. A case report and review of the literature. J Cardiovasc Surg 2001;42:237–240.

57. Jhirad R, Kalman PG. Mycotic axillary artery aneurysm. J Vasc Surg 1998;28:708–709.

58. Wilson WR, Lie JT, Houser OW, et al. The management of patients with mycotic aneurysms. Curr Clin Top Infect Dis 1981;2:151–183.

59. Mansur AJ, Grinberg M, Leao PP, et al. Extracranial mycotic aneurysms in infective endocarditis. Clin Cardiol 1986;9:65–72.

60. Reece IJ, al Tareif H, Tolia J, Saeed FA. Mycotic aneurysm of the left anterior descending coronary artery after aortic endocarditis. A case report and brief review of the literature. Tex Heart Inst J 1994;21:231–235.

61. Krapf H, Skalej M, Voight K. Subarachnoid hemorrhage due to septic embolic infarction in infective endocarditis. Cerebrovasc Dis 1999;9:182–184.

62. Bohmfalk GL, Story JL, Wissinger JP, Brown WE Jr. Bacterial intracranial aneurysm. J Neurosurg 1978;48:369–382.

63. Roach MR, Drake CG. Ruptured cerebral aneurysms caused by microorganisms. N Engl J Med 1965;273:240–244.

64. Cosmo LY, Risi G, Nelson S, et al. Fatal hemoptysis in acute bacterial endocarditis. Am Rev Respir Dis 1988;137:1223–1226.

65. Camarata PJ, Latchaw RE, Rufenacht DA, Heros RC. Intracranial aneurysms. Invest Radiol 1993;28:373–382.

66. Lerner P. Neurologic complications of infective endocarditis. Med Clin North Am 1985;69:385–398.

67. Clare CE, Barrow DL. Infectious intracranial aneurysms. Neurosurg Clin N Am 1992;3:551–566.

68. Huston J III, Nichols DA, Luetmer PH, et al. Blinded prospective evaluation of sensitivity of MR angiography to known intracranial aneurysms: importance of aneurysm size. Am J Neuroradiol 1994;15:1607–1614.

69. McKinsey DS, McMurray TI, Flynn JM. Immune complex glomerulonephritis associated with *Staphylococcus aureus* bacteremia: response to corticosteroid therapy. Rev Infect Dis 1990;12:125–127.

70. Eknoyan G, Lister BJ, Kim HS, Greenberg SD. Renal complications of bacterial endocarditis. Am J Nephrol 1985;5:457–469.

71. Weinstein L, Schlesinger JJ. Pathoanatomic, pathophysiologic and clinical correlations in endocarditis. N Engl J Med 1974;291:832–837.

72. Roberts-Thomson PJ, Rischmueller M, Kwiatek RA, et al. Rheumatic manifestations of infective endocarditis. Rheumatol Int 1992;12:61–63.

73. Churchill MA Jr., Geraci JE, Hunder GG. Musculoskeletal manifestations of bacterial endocarditis. Ann Intern Med 1977;87:754–759.

74. Yee J, McAllister CK. The utility of Osler's nodes in the diagnosis of infective endocarditis. Chest 1987;92:751–752.

75. Watanakunakorn C. Osler's nodes on the dorsum of the foot. Chest 1988;94:1088–1090.

76. Alpert JS, Krous HF, Dalen JE, et al. Pathogenesis of Osler's nodes. Ann Intern Med 1976;85:471–473.

77. Barham NJ, Flint EJ, Mifsud RP. Osteomyelitis complicating *Streptococcus milleri* endocarditis. Postgrad Med J 1990;66:314–315.

78. Nightingale AK, Kuo J, Ring NJ, Marshall AJ. A case of mitral valve endocarditis complicated by cerebral infarction and lumbar discitis. Br J Cardiol 2001;8:246–248.

79. Pascaretti C, Legrand E, Laporte J, et al. Bacterial endocarditis revealed by infectious discitis. Rev Rhum Engl Ed 1996;63:119–123.

80. Pruitt AA, Rubin RH, Karchmer AW, Duncan GW. Neurologic complications of bacterial endocarditis. Medicine 1978;57:329–343.

81. Robbins MJ, Soeiro R, Frishman WH, Strom JA. Right-sided valvular endocarditis: etiology, diagnosis and an approach to therapy. Am Heart J 1986;111:128–135.

82. Cassling RS, Rogler WC, McManus BM. Isolated pulmonic valve infective endocarditis: a diagnostically elusive entity. Am Heart J 1985;109:558–567.

83. Dressler FA, Roberts WC. Infective endocarditis in opiate addicts: analysis of 80 cases studied at necropsy. Am J Cardiol 1989;63:1240–1257.

84. Sexauer WP, Quezado Z, Lippmann ML, Goldberg SK. Pleural effusions in right-sided endocarditis: characteristics and pathophysiology. South Med J 1992;85:1176–1180.

85. Federmann M, Dirsch OR, Jenni R. Pacemaker endocarditis. Heart 1996;75:446.

86. Tang DC, Huang TP. Internal jugular vein haemodialysis catheter-induced right atrial endocarditis—case report and review of literature. Scand J Urol Nephrol 1998;32:411–414.

87. Hecht SR, Berger M. Right sided endocarditis in intravenous drug users. Ann Intern Med 1992;117:560–566.

88. Chambers HF, Morris DL, Tauber MG, Modin G. Cocaine use and the risk for endocarditis in intravenous drug users. Ann Intern Med 1987;106:833–836.

89. Cacoub P, Leprince P, Nataf P, et al. Pacemaker infective endocarditis. Am J Cardiol 1998;82:480–484.

90. Miralles A, Moncada V, Chevez H, et al. Pacemaker endocarditis: approach for lead extraction in endocarditis with large vegetations. Ann Thorac Surg 2001;72:2130–2132.

91. Chu JJ, Lin PT, Chang CH, et al. Video-assisted endoscopic removal of infected pacemaker lead with large floating vegetations. Pacing Clin Electrophysiol 1999;22:1700–1703.

92. Naggar CZ, Forgacs P. Infective endocarditis: a challenging disease. Med Clin North Am 1986;70:1279–1294.

93. Griffin MR, Wilson WR, Edwards WD, et al. Infective endocarditis—Olmstead County, Minnesota, 1950 through 1981. JAMA 1985;254:1199–1202.

94. Arvay A, Lengyel M. Incidence and risk factors of prosthetic valve endocarditis. Eur J Cardiothorac Surg 1988;2:340–346.

95. Bortolotti U, Thiene G, Milano A, et al. Pathological study of infective endocarditis on Hancock porcine bioprostheses. J Thorac Cardiovasc Surg 1981;81:934–942.

96. Horstkotte D, Korfer R, Loogen F, et al. Prosthetic valve endocarditis: clinical findings and management. Eur Heart J 1984;5(Suppl C):117–122.

97. Chastre J, Trouillet JL. Early infective endocarditis in prosthetic valves. Eur Heart J 1995;16(Suppl B):32–38.

98. John MD, Hibberd PL, Marchmer AS, et al. *Staphylococcus aureus* prosthetic valve endocarditis: optimal management and risk factors for death. Clin Infect Dis 1998;26:1302–1309.

99. Braunwald E. Infective endocarditis. In: Heart Disease. A Textbook of Cardiovascular Medicine, 4th edn. WB Saunders; 1992:1082.

100. de Gevigney G, Pop C, Delahaye JP. The risk of infective endocarditis after cardiac surgical and interventional procedures. Eur Heart J 1995;16:(Suppl B):7–14.

101. Horstkotte D, Piper C, Niehues R, et al. Late prosthetic valve endocarditis. Eur Heart J 1995;16(Suppl B):39–47.

102. Rubinstein E, Lang R. Fungal endocarditis. Eur Heart J 1995;16(Suppl B):84–89.

103. Moyer DV, Edwards Jr JE. Fungal endocarditis. In: Kaye D, ed. Infective endocarditis, 2nd edn. New York: Raven Press; 1992:299–312.

104. McLeod R, Remington JS. Fungal endocarditis. In: Rahimtoola SH et al, eds. Infective Endocarditis. New York: Grune & Stratton; 1978:211–290.

105. Kammer RB, Utz JP. *Aspergillus* species endocarditis: the face of a not so rare disease. Am J Med 1974;56:506–521.

106. Seelig MS, Speth CP, Kozinn PJ, et al. Patterns of *Candida* endocarditis following cardiac surgery: importance of early diagnosis and therapy (an analysis of 91 cases). Prog Cardiovasc Dis 1974;17:125–160.

107. Rubinstein E, Noriega ER, Simberkoff MS, Holzman R, Rahal Jr JJ. Fungal endocarditis: analysis of 24 cases and review of the literature. Medicine 1975;54:331–344.

108. Microbiology Resource Committee, College of American Pathologists. Memorandum to CAP Mycology Survey participants re 1987 Survey set F-B. Traverse City, Michigan, 1987.

109. Paya CV, Roberts GD, Cockerill RF. Laboratory methods for the diagnosis of disseminated histoplasmosis. Mayo Clinic Proc 1987;62:480–485.

110. Bisbe J, Miro JM, Torres JM, et al. Diagnostic value of serum antibody and antigen detection in heroin addicts with systemic candidiasis. Rev Infect Dis 1989;11:310–315.

111. Weiner MH. Antigenaemia detected by radioimmunoassay in systemic aspergillosis. Ann Intern Med 1980;92:793–796.

112. Donal E, Abgueguen P, Coisne D, et al. Echocardiographic features of *Candida* species endocarditis: 12 cases and a review of published reports. Heart 2001;86:179–182.

113. Lengyel M. The impact of transesophageal echocardiography on the management of prosthetic valve endocarditis: experience of 31 cases and review of the literature. J Heart Valve Dis 1997;6:204–211.

114. Walsh TJ, Hutchins GM, Bulkley BH, et al. Fungal infections of the heart: analysis of 51 autopsy cases. Am J Cardiol 1980;45:357–366.

115. Andriole VT, Kravetz HM, Roberts WC, et al. *Candida* endocarditis. Am J Med 1962;32:251–285.

116. Gregg CR, McGee ZA, Bodner SJ, et al. Fungal endocarditis complicating treatment of prosthetic valve bacterial endocarditis: value of prophylactic oral nystatin. South Med J 1987;80:1407–1409.

117. Oakley CM. The medical treatment of culture-negative infective endocarditis. Eur Heart J 1995;16(Suppl B):39–47.

118. Brouqui P, Raoult D. Endocarditis due to rare and fastidious bacteria. Clin Microbiol Rev 2001;14:177–207.

119. Rolain JM, Maurin M, Raoult D. Bactericidal effect of antibiotics on *Bartonella* and *Brucella* spp.: clinical complications. J Antimicrob Chemother 2000;46:811–814.

120. Popat K, Barnardo D, Webb-Peploe M. *Mycoplasma pneumoniae* endocarditis. Br Heart J 1980;44:111–112.

121. Al-Kasab S, al-Fagih MR, al-Yousef S, et al. *Brucella* infective endocarditis. Successful combined medical and surgical therapy. J Thorac Cardiovasc Surg 1988;95:862–867.

122. Shafer RW, Braverman ER. Q-fever endocarditis: delay in diagnosis due to an apparent clinical response to corticosteroids. Am J Med 1989;86:729.

123. Jones RB, Priest JB, Kuo C. Subacute chlamydial endocarditis. JAMA 1982;247:655–658.

124. Fernandez-Guerrero ML, Muelas JM, Aguado JM, et al. Q-fever endocarditis on porcine bioprosthetic valves. Clinicopathologic features and microbiologic findings in three patients with doxycycline, cotrimoxazole and valve replacement. Ann Intern Med 1988;108;209–213.

125. Brearley BF, Hutchinson DN. Endocarditis associated with *Chlamydia trachomatis* infection. Br Heart J 1981;46:220–221.

126. Noseda A, Liesnard C, Goffin Y, Thys JP. Q-fever endocarditis: relapse 5 years after successful valve replacement for a first unrecognized episode. J Cardiovasc Surg 1988;29:360–363.

127. Stein A, Raoult D. Q fever endocarditis. Eur Heart J 1985;16(Suppl B):19–23.

128. Cohen JI, Sloss LJ, Kundsin R, Golightly L. Prosthetic valve endocarditis caused by *Mycoplasma hominis*. Am J Med 1989;86:819–821.

129. Demiricin M, Dogan R, Peker O, et al. Aortic insufficiency and enterococcal endocarditis complicating systemic lupus erythematosus. Thorac Cardiovasc Surg 1995;43:302–304.

130. Houpikian P, Habib G, Mesana T, Raoult D. Changing clinical presentation of Q fever endocarditis. Clin Infect Dis 2000;34:E 28–31.

131. Musso D, Raoult D. *Coxiella burnetii* blood cultures from acute and chronic Q-fever patients. J Clin Microbiol 1995;33:3129–3132.

132. Akinci E, Gol MK, Balbay Y. A case of prosthetic mitral valve endocarditis caused by *Brucella abortus*. Scand Infect Dis 2001;33:71–72.

133. Raoult D, Urvolgyi J, Etienne J, et al. Diagnosis of endocarditis in acute Q-fever by immunofluorescence serology. Acta Virol 1988;32:70–74.

134. Fournier PE. Diagnosis of Q fever. J Clin Microbiol 1998;36:1823–1834.

135. Peacock MG. Serological evaluation of Q fever in humans: enhanced phase 1 titres of immunoglobulins G and A are diagnostic for Q fever endocarditis. Infect Immun 1983;41:1089–1098.

136. Tissot-Dupont H. Q fever serology: cutoff determination for microimmunofluorescence. Clin Diag Lab Immunol 1994;1:189–196.

137. Siegman-Igra Y, Kaufman O, Kaysary A, et al. Q-fever endocarditis in Israel and a worldwide review. Scand J Infect Dis 1997;29:41–49.

138. Raoult D, Fournier PE, Drancourt M, et al. Diagnosis of 22 new cases of *Bartonella* endocarditis. Ann Intern Med 1996;125:646–652.

139. Brouqui P. Immunohistologic demonstration of *Coxiella burnetii* in the valves of patients with Q fever endocarditis. Am J Med 1994;97:451–458.

140. Muhlemann K, Matter L, Meyer B, et al. Isolation of *Coxiella burnetii* from heart valves of patients treated for Q-fever endocarditis. J Clin Microbiol 1995;33:428–431.

141. Raoult D. Monoclonal antibodies to *Coxiella burnetii* for antigenic detection in cell cultures and in paraffin embedded tissues. Am J Clin Pathol 1994;101:318–320.

142. Etienne J, Ory D, Thouvenot D, et al. Chlamydial endocarditis: a report of 10 cases. Eur Heart J 1992;13:1422–1426.

143. Woods GL. Detection of infection or infectious agents by use of cytologic and histologic stains. Clin Microbiol Rev 1996;9:382–404.

144. Goldenberger D, Künzli A, Vogt P, et al. Molecular diagnosis of bacterial endocarditis by broad-range PCR amplification and direct sequencing. J Clin Microbiol 1997;35:2733–2739.

145. Stein A. Detection of *Coxiella burnetii* by DNA amplification using polymerase chain reaction. J Clin Microbiol 1992;30:2462–2466.

146. Ramzan NN, Loftus E Jr., Burgart LJ, et al. Diagnosis and monitoring of Whipple's disease by polymerase chain reaction. Ann Intern Med 1997;126:520–527.

147. Nikkari S, Gotoff R, Bourbeau PP, et al. Identification of *Cardiobacterium hominis* by broad-range bacterial polymerase chain reaction analysis in a case of culture-negative endocarditis. Arch Intern Med 2002;162:477–479.

148. Lisby G, Gutschik E, Durack DT. Molecular methods for diagnosis of infective endocarditis. Infect Dis Clin North Am 2002;16:393–412.

149. Fournier P-E, Raoult D. Nonculture laboratory methods for the diagnosis of infectious endocarditis. Current Science 1999;1:136–141.

CHAPTER 3

Investigations

Mild to moderate anemia is commonly present in IE with a normochromic, normocytic picture. Neutrophil leukocytosis is common and the erythrocyte sedimentation rate (ESR) and C-reactive protein (CRP) are elevated in 90% of patients and the latter have been proposed as additional minor criteria to the Duke classification of IE [1–4]. Intraleukocyte bacteria can be seen in buffy coat preparations of blood in up to 50% of cases [5].

Urine examination may reveal microscopic hematuria and/or proteinuria in 50% of cases. In those developing immune complex glomerulonephritis, red blood cell casts and heavy proteinuria may be identified. Renal function should be repeatedly monitored to detect dysfunction early. A polyclonal increase in gammaglobulins is characteristic of active endocarditis and an elevated rheumatoid factor may be of diagnostic help [6,7].

Blood cultures remain the definitive procedure for diagnosing IE [8]. At least three sets of blood cultures (aerobic and anaerobic) drawn >1 hour apart should be taken and if positive for the same organism (in the majority of the culture bottles), this confirms that an endovascular infection is likely. Although IE caused by anaerobes is uncommon, blood cultures should be incubated in both aerobic and anaerobic conditions in an attempt to detect organisms such as *Clostridium* or *Bacteroides* species.

An ECG and chest X-ray are useful for assessing the extent and severity of the infection, its effects on cardiac size and function, and for determining whether surgery needs to be considered early or whether prophylactic temporary pacemaker implantation is indicated. The presence of significant conduction abnormalities demonstrated on the ECG (Figure 3.1), especially if known to be new or progressive, warrants urgent temporary pacing and this is classically seen in the presence of aortic root abscesses complicating aortic valve endocarditis due to *Staphylococcus aureus* infection [9–12] (Figures 3.2 and 3.3). Arrhythmias may be caused by myocarditis or by ischemia due to coronary emboli and should be treated in standard fashion.

A chest X-ray may show evidence of cardiomegaly and heart failure (Figures 3.4–3.6) but in tricuspid valve endocarditis in intravenous drug abusers (Figures 3.7–3.9) or in patients with serious permanent pacemaker infection it may demonstrate infective pulmonary emboli and pulmonary abscesses (Figures 3.10 and 3.11). Computer-assisted tomography (CAT) scanning may help confirm a suspicious pulmonary shadow to be an abscess (Figure 3.12) and even identify embolization of vegetations into the pulmonary circulation (Figures 3.13–3.15). The presence of a splenic abscess in a patient with splenomegaly (Figure 3.16) may also be confirmed by CAT scanning.

CAT scanning is an essential investigation of intracranial pathology. It distinguishes between hemorrhage, infarction, and abscess by their different X-ray attenuation. Hemorrhage typically produces a high attenuation image, infarction a low attenuation image, and an abscess a low area of attenuation surrounded by a high attenuation ring (see Figures 2.26–2.28).

Infection-related antiphospholipid antibodies may be helpful in predicting risk of embolic events and the application of polymerase chain reaction (PCR) technology to blood and tissue samples may be useful for identifying more unusual pathogens causing IE [13–17].

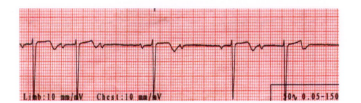

FIGURE 3.1 Complete heart block may complicate infective endocarditis involving the interventricular septum often with abscess formation. Intracardiac pacing is indicated as an emergency. Courtesy of Dr Chris Bellamy.

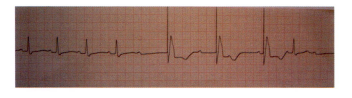

FIGURE 3.2 Temporary pacing from epicardial pacing wires is essential postoperatively in patients with conduction defects associated with prosthetic aortic valve endocarditis and paravalvular abscess due to *Staphylococcus aureus*.

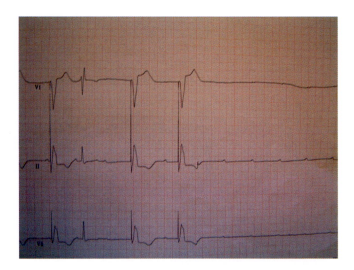

FIGURE 3.3 Switching off the temporary pacemaker shows the underlying rhythm to be complete heart block with ventricular standstill and permanent pacemaker implantation is usually necessary.

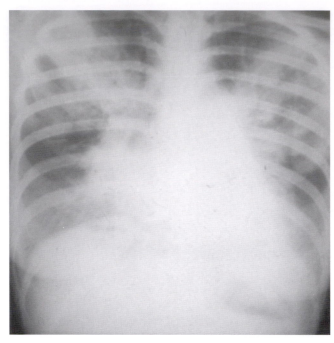

FIGURE 3.4 Chest X-ray showing cardiomegaly and pulmonary edema due to severe aortic regurgitation as a result of *Staphylococcus aureus* endocarditis affecting the aortic valve.

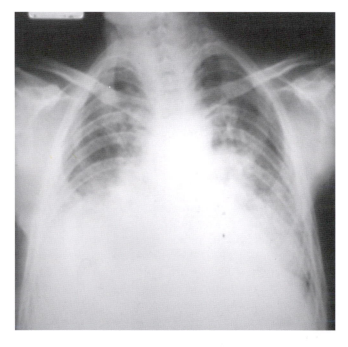

FIGURE 3.5 Chest X-ray showing pulmonary edema due to acute mitral regurgitation as a result of *Staphylococcus aureus* induced mitral valve endocarditis.

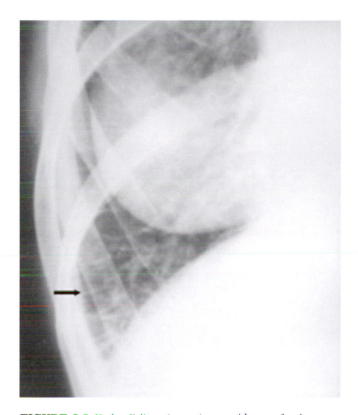

FIGURE 3.6 Kerley B lines (arrow) are evidence of pulmonary edema.

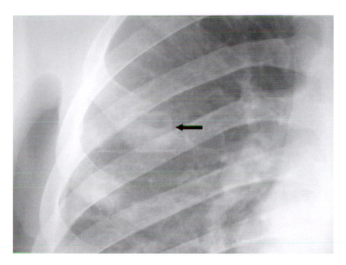

FIGURE 3.8 A magnified view of an abscess cavity (arrow). Courtesy of Dr Hilary Fewins.

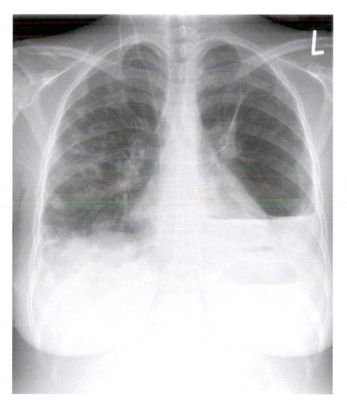

FIGURE 3.9 Chest X-ray showing many of the features typical of right-sided infective endocarditis complicated by septic pulmonary emboli. Multiple alveolar opacities are noted in the right lung. Abscess formation in the left lung has caused a bronchopleural fistula, pneumothorax, and empyema, hence the fluid level. The patient has a central intravascular catheter placed for antibiotic administration. Courtesy of Dr Brad Munt and Dr Rob Moss. Heart 2003;89:577–581. Reproduced with permission from the BMJ Publishing Group.

FIGURE 3.7 Chest X-ray showing multiple pulmonary abscesses in a 26-year-old IV drug abuser with *Staphylococcus aureus* infective endocarditis on the tricuspid valve. A typical appearance of a rounded opacity with air and fluid level (arrow) is characteristic of an abscess.

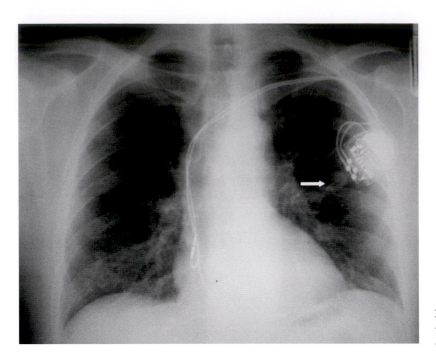

FIGURE 3.10 Chest X-ray in a patient with pyrexia 4 years after dual chamber pacemaker implantation. An opacity is visible in the left upper lobe (arrow).

When valve replacement is undertaken, valvular tissue (including vegetations) should be examined histologically and cultured for the presence of organisms, which may allow postoperative antibiotics to be tailored accordingly. Bacterial DNA probe analysis of explanted tissue and amplification by PCR may be an alternative to histology and culture.

The key tests, however, are blood cultures and echocardiography.

OPTIMAL BLOOD CULTURE TECHNIQUE

Between three and six sets of blood cultures should be obtained at intervals > 1 hour within the first 24 hours from all patients suspected of having IE before commencing antibiotic treatment (Figure 3.17).

Three sets of blood cultures should be taken if the patient is extremely unwell and the clinical features suggest

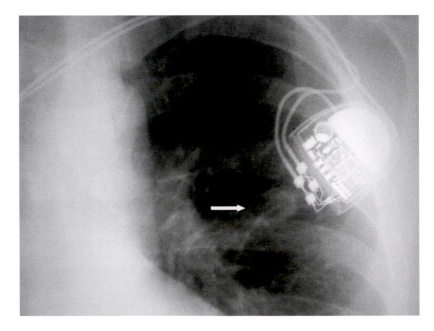

FIGURE 3.11 Close-up view of the opacity shown in Figure 3.10 suggests that this may be an abscess. Blood cultures demonstrated *Staphylococcus aureus.*

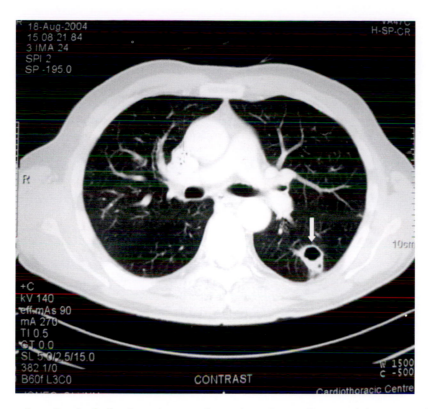

FIGURE 3.12 CAT scan confirms that the shadow is a pulmonary abscess (arrow). A smaller second abscess was identified in the right upper lobe.

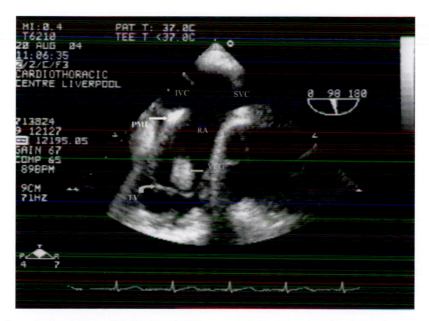

FIGURE 3.13 Transesophageal echocardiography demonstrated a 1 cm vegetation on a tricuspid valve leaflet. The pacing system was removed under local anesthetic whilst the patient was treated with IV flucloxacillin 3 g four times a day. A temporary pacemaker was not placed as the original indication was sick sinus syndrome and sinus arrest. IVC, inferior vena cava; SVC, superior vena cava; RA, right atrium; TV, tricuspid valve; VEG, vegetation; PML, pacemaker lead.

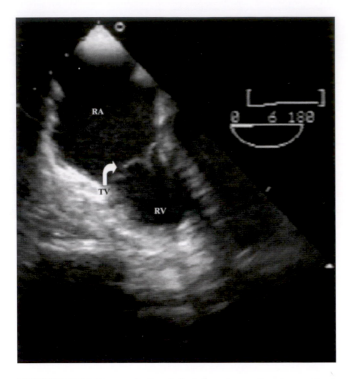

FIGURE 3.14 Removal of an infected pacing system in a patient with a vegetation on the tricuspid valve may result in embolization of the vegetation into the pulmonary circulation. This repeat TEE in the same patient shown in Figure 3.13 reveals that the vegetation has disappeared from the tricuspid valve. RA, right atrium; RV, right ventricle; TV, tricuspid valve.

that endocarditis is very likely and six sets if the patient is not acutely ill or when the diagnosis is not obvious clinically. Optimal aseptic technique is necessary when taking the blood cultures to avoid missing the diagnosis as well as to avoid false positive cases due to contaminating organisms from the skin [18,19]. Each set of blood cultures should be taken via a separate venepuncture (10 ml of blood into each bottle).

The bacteremia associated with IE is typically continuous, with 10–200 colony-forming units per milliliter of blood [20]. However, this is not always the case and some patients may have intermittent bacteremia or less than one organism per milliliter of blood. In such cases, the number of positive culture results is directly related to the number of blood samples drawn and the volume of blood in each individual sample. Single samples should not be drawn because the most common contaminants, coagulase-negative staphylococci, can be responsible for endocarditis and a positive culture will be difficult to interpret [21]. Ideally, cultures should be spaced at least 60 minutes apart to prove that bacteremia is continuous. Blood cultures should be stored in an incubator at 37°C and not in a refrigerator (Figure 3.18). The possibility of IE should be made clear on the request form (Figure 3.19).

Overall, about two-thirds of all samples drawn from patients with IE are positive (Figures 3.20 and 3.21). Those patients with untreated endocarditis and continuous bacteremia will generally have positive culture results in all samples [22]. Ninety percent will be diagnosed by the first sample and 95% after three cultures [21–23]. Other patients will have a much lower incidence of positive cultures. These include patients who have already received antibiotic treatment, those with fungal endocarditis or with "difficult-to-culture" organisms, and those with CNE [24]. It has been estimated that blood cultures may be negative in as many as 25% of patients who received recent outpatient antibiotic therapy [25–28] and it may be prudent to delay treatment (dependent on clinical status of patient) in order to maximize the chance of obtaining positive blood cultures. Culturing arterial rather than venous blood and drawing blood during spikes of temperature do not appear to be of any additional value [29]. When blood cultures are negative because of previous antibiotic therapy, the period of time required for the blood cultures to become positive again varies from 24 hours to 2 weeks depending on the activity of the antibiotic against the organism and the duration of prior treatment. If treatment has been received for only 2–3 days, cultures will probably revert to positive quickly. It is important to indicate on the request form whether antibiotics have been received by the patient so that special culture methods for unusual organisms, lysis centrifugation techniques, or serology may be considered. Identification should be to species level.

The yield of positive cultures of "slow-growing" organisms, such as nutritionally variant streptococci (approximately 5% of streptococci in IE) and the fastidious Gram-negative aerobic bacilli such as *Haemophilus* spp. or *Bartonella* spp., may be improved by prolonged incubation

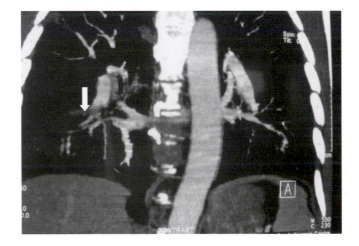

FIGURE 3.15 A CAT scan shows the vegetation to have embolized into a branch of the right lower pulmonary artery (arrow).

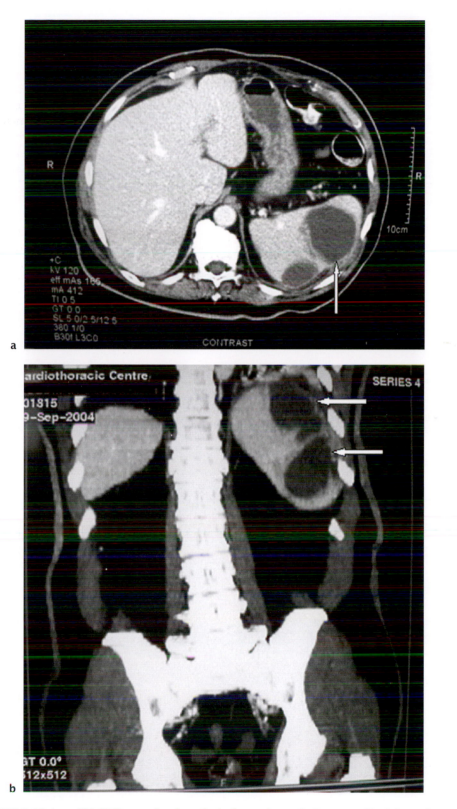

FIGURE 3.16 (**a** and **b**) CAT scans showing splenic abscess (arrows). Courtesy of Dr John Holemans.

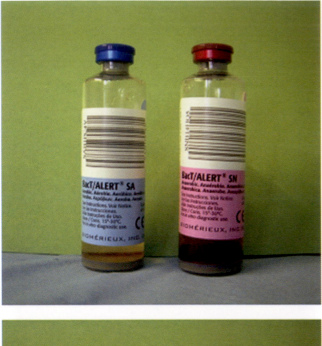

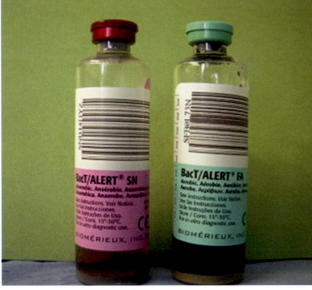

FIGURE 3.17 10 ml of blood needs to be added to both aerobic and anaerobic blood culture bottles. The top illustration shows the bottles to be used when a patient is not on antibiotic treatment and the bottom illustration, the bottles to be used if the patient has already received antibiotics. The culture media in the latter bottles contain charcoal resin to remove antibiotic from the blood.

(7–21 days) (e.g. on chocolate agar plates) or by using optimized blood culture media [30–34]. The microbiology laboratory should be informed when such organisms are suspected. Serum can be analyzed for antibodies against organisms that cannot be cultured routinely or antibodies to Gram-positive bacterial cell walls. PCR may also be

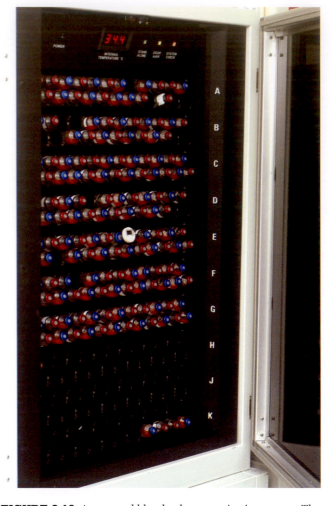

FIGURE 3.18 Automated blood culture monitoring system. The pairs of blood culture bottles are loaded directly into this incubator/detector as soon as possible after being collected. Continuous monitoring allows the earliest detection of bacterial growth. Courtesy of Dr Mike Rothburn.

applied to blood samples or the original growth-negative blood culture substrate.

ECHOCARDIOGRAPHY

Echocardiography is the most useful tool for confirming the anatomical diagnosis, e.g. hypertrophic obstructive cardiomyopathy and mitral valve prolapse (Figures 3.22 and 3.23) and for demonstrating vegetations on valves or other structures [35–41] (Figures 3.24 and 3.25). It should be performed by appropriately trained personnel accredited in echocardiography (Figure 3.26).

M-mode transthoracic echocardiography (TTE) has been used for the detection of vegetations associated with

DIAGNOSTIC REQUEST (NON-UROGENITAL)
The Royal Liverpool and Broadgreen University Hospitals NHS Trust
Enquiries Telephone 0151 706 4410/1
Date: 4/1/04
Time: 13.50pm
Urgent phoned result required on extension: 2388
Unit No 123456A
Surname OTHER
Forenames ARTHUR N
Date of Birth 22.10.35 M/F M
Relevant clinical details PYREXIA / Unwell FINGER Clubbing AORTIC REGURGITATION ?INFECTIVE ENDOCARDITIS
Is TB suspected: Yes / No ☑
Antibiotics: Recent / Current / Planned ☑
Pregnant: Yes / No ☑
Requesting M.O.: (Please print) D. RAMSDALE
Bleep number: 2371
Ward / Clinic: A Hospital: CTC
Consultant: D. RAMSDALE NHS / Private
BACTERIOLOGY
NON-UROGENITAL SWABS
CONJUCTIVAL: Left / Right / Both
CORNEAL TISSUE: Left / Right
THROAT
WOUND
PUS
BIOPSY
LINE TIP
OTHER SWAB
BLOOD CULTURES, FLUIDS & ASSAYS
☑ BLOOD CULTURE
FLUID
CSF
ASCITIC
DIALYSATE
Joint:
Other:
ANTIBIOTICS ASSAY
Predose
Drug: Postdose
Dosage: Check for clearance
SPUTUM / BAL / TRACHEAL ASP
Routine
TB
Other investigation:
FAECES
Routine
Ova / Cysts / Parasites
OTHER
Mycology examination
TB culture
OTHER Please state specimen & request
CPA ACCREDITED

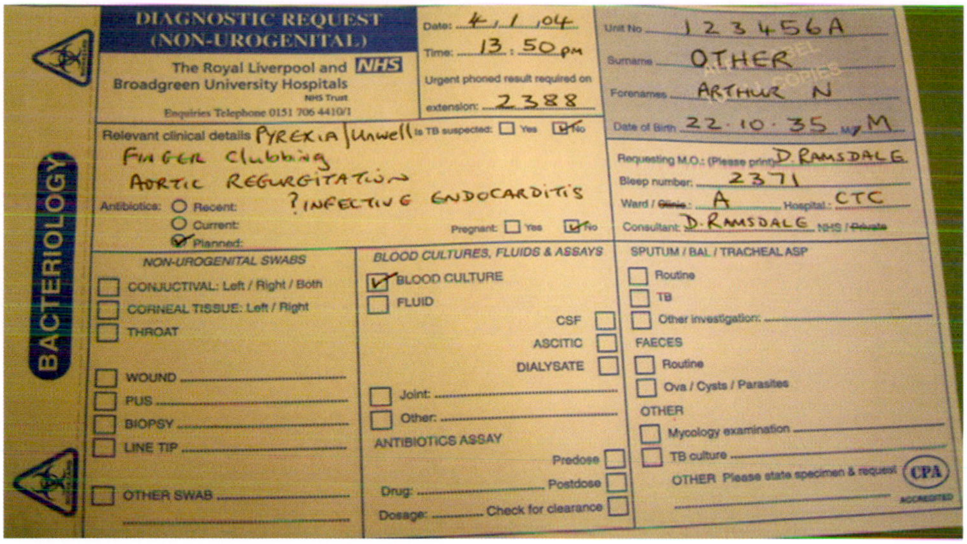

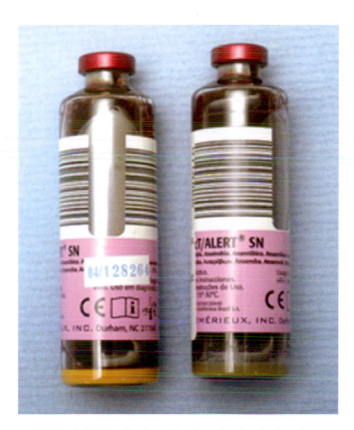

FIGURE 3.19 Request forms should be fully completed accurately and legibly and as much clinical information as possible should be provided. Specimens should be placed in an incubator without delay and not refrigerated overnight.

IE since 1973 (Figure 3.27) and 2-D echocardiography since 1977 (Figures 3.28 and 3.29). Reports suggest a specificity of 98% and a sensitivity of 60–75% and echocardiography should be performed early in all patients clinically suspected of having IE, including those with negative blood cultures [42–48]. However, vegetation size affects sensitivity and it has been suggested that although 70% of vegetations between 6 and 10 mm are identified, only 25% of those <5 mm are recognized [37]. Cardiac myxomas can present with pyrexia and a new cardiac murmur but transthoracic echocardiography can distinguish

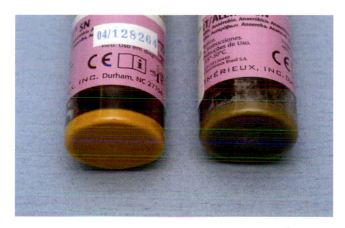

FIGURE 3.20 Blood culture bottles after incubation showing color change in positive bottle indicating the need for subculture onto agar plates for identification tests and antibiotic susceptibility. In culture-negative endocarditis, the bottles do not signal as positive. Courtesy of Dr Mike Rothburn.

FIGURE 3.21 Blood culture bottle showing positive result (left—color changes from green to yellow) typically within 18 hours incubation at 37°C. The growth of bacteria is detected by production of carbon dioxide and by a pH sensor at the base of the bottle. The color change is detected by continuous reading by a colorimeter. Courtesy of Dr Mike Rothburn.

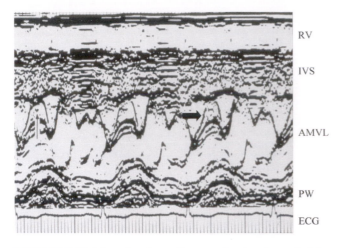

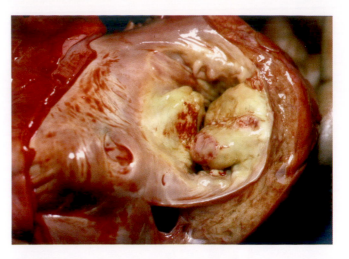

FIGURE 3.22 M-mode echocardiogram showing the typical features of hypertrophic obstructive cardiomyopathy, including asymmetric hypertrophy of the interventricular septum (IVS) and systolic anterior movement of the mitral valve (SAM) (arrow). RV, right ventricle; AMVL, anterior mitral valve leaflet; PW, posterior wall of left ventricle; ECG, electrocardiogram.

FIGURE 3.25 Vegetations on both anterior and posterior mitral valve leaflets can usually be identified by echocardiography.

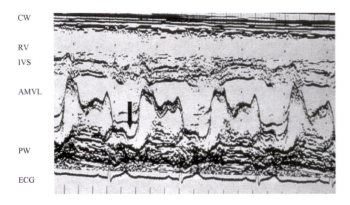

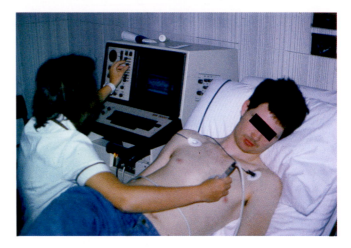

FIGURE 3.23 M-mode echocardiogram in mitral valve prolapse showing posterior prolapse of the mitral valve (arrow). CW, chest wall; RV, right ventricle; IVS, interventricular septum; AMVL, anterior mitral valve leaflet; PW, posterior wall of left ventricle; ECG, electrocardiogram.

FIGURE 3.26 Transthoracic echocardiogram being performed.

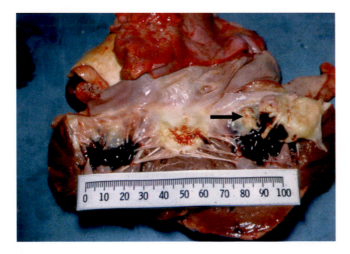

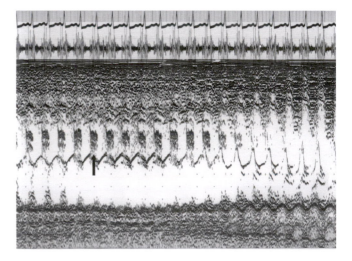

FIGURE 3.24 Myxomatous mitral valve infected with vegetations (arrow).

FIGURE 3.27 M-mode transthoracic echocardiogram showing aortic valve vegetations (arrow).

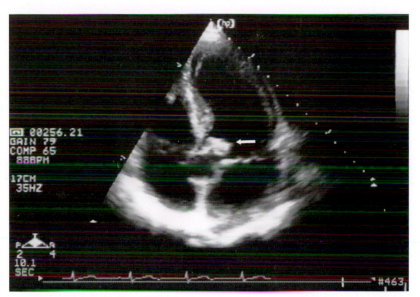

FIGURE 3.28 2-D transthoracic echocardiogram showing large pedunculated vegetation (arrow) on the aortic valve due to *Enterococcus faecalis* endocarditis.

between vegetations and myxoma (Figures 3.30 and 3.31). Myxomas are often fragile, may embolize and should be removed surgically (Figures 3.32 and 3.33).

Transesophageal echocardiography (TEE), initially described in the late 1980s, has proved most valuable in assessing patients with suspected endocarditis—being more sensitive (95%) than transthoracic echocardiography for detecting and sizing vegetations, abscesses, pseudoaneurysms, and valvular perforations [37–53] (Figure 3.34). The absolute sensitivity depends upon the site and the size of the abnormalities [40,54–56]. TEE is usually performed under sedation (Figures 3.35–3.40).

TEE using biplanar and multiplanar probes with color flow, continuous and pulse-wave Doppler is more sensitive than TTE for detecting abscesses in patients with both NVE and PVE (87% versus 28%) [57–60]. TEE is the technique of choice in evaluating a patient with suspected PVE (since it is more likely to demonstrate a perivalvular abscess, dehiscence, and fistulas) (Figure 3.41), for those with NVE who have a prolonged course of infection, for those with endocarditis at unusual sites e.g. pacemaker leads, and for those who do not respond to adequate medical therapy [37,52,57–65]. TEE is perhaps more useful in tissue rather than mechanical PVE as it is often difficult to see detail on mechanical valves because of intense interfering echoes from the metal struts and valve ring [66].

Echocardiography may not only demonstrate vegetations (Figure 3.42), fistulas, valve perforations,

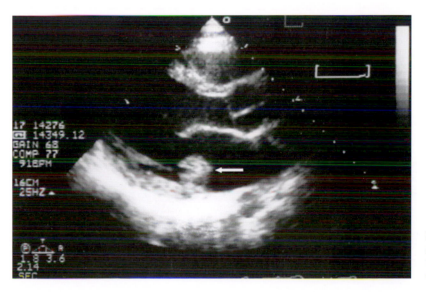

FIGURE 3.29 2-D transthoracic echocardiogram showing large vegetation on posterior leaflet of mitral valve (arrow) in a patient with *Streptococcus mitis* endocarditis.

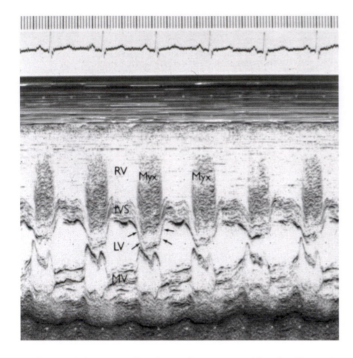

FIGURE 3.30 M-mode echocardiogram provides the diagnosis of a rare right atrial myxoma which prolapses through the tricuspid valve. RV, right ventricle; Myx, myxoma; MV, mitral valve; IVS, interventricular septum; LV, left ventricle.

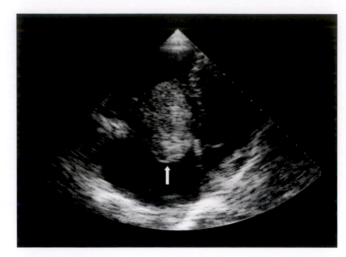

FIGURE 3.31 2-D echocardiogram confirms the M-mode suggestion of large right atrial myxoma (arrow) which prolapses across the tricuspid valve and into the right ventricle and excludes the possibility of tricuspid valve vegetations.

pseudoaneurysms, perivalvular complications such as abscesses (Figures 3.43–3.47) and predict embolic risk in IE but it also provides information on left ventricular function and an estimate of severity of regurgitant flow [67–70] (Figures 3.48–3.53). Premature mitral valve closure in acute aortic regurgitation suggests the need for urgent surgical intervention. Repeat echocardiography is often useful

for early detection of cardiac complications requiring surgical intervention.

Using continuous wave Doppler, systolic high velocity flow suggests an abnormal communication between the aorta and either the left or right atria and using color Doppler, the site of fistulous communications may be well defined (Figure 3.54).

For suspected NVE, a TTE should be the initial echo study. If the TTE is technically inadequate, then a TEE should be performed. If the TTE is clearly positive or clearly negative, no further echo is necessary, although the diagnosis of IE cannot be excluded. However, a TEE should be performed if the TTE is abnormal but nondiagnostic.

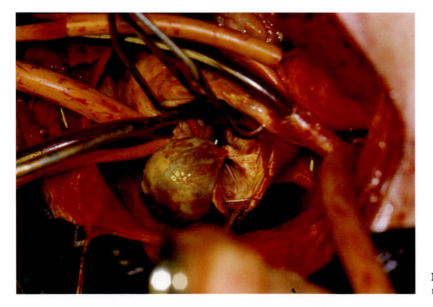

FIGURE 3.32 Open heart surgery is necessary to remove myxomas.

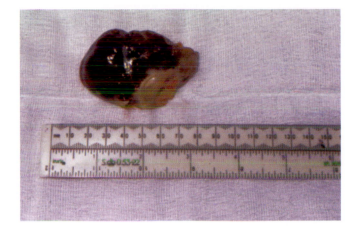

FIGURE 3.33 Myxoma removed from right atrium. Once removed and devoid of blood supply, the tumors often appear to "shrink" in size.

CARDIAC CATHETERIZATION IN INFECTIVE ENDOCARDITIS

Doppler echocardiography allows accurate assessment of the hemodynamic and pathological consequences of infection in most cases. The use of invasive techniques is usually limited to coronary arteriography in those with a history of angina or risk factors for coronary artery disease and to aortography for the identification of sinus of Valsalva aneurysms (Figure 3.55), the severity of aortic regurgitation (Figure 3.56), or fistulous connections between chambers if echocardiography is inconclusive. Left ventricular (LV) angiography will demonstrate LV

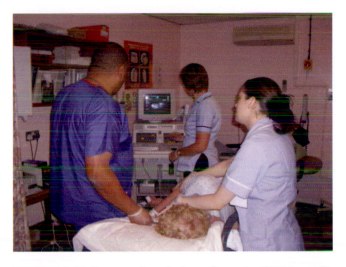

FIGURE 3.35 Transesophageal echocardiography (TEE) is usually performed under sedation. A cardiologist, an echocardiographer, and a nurse are usually necessary. Courtesy of Dr Serge Osula and Dr Malcolm Burgess.

function and the presence and severity of mitral regurgitation (Figure 3.57). The latter may also be indicated by the large "V" wave in a pulmonary capillary wedge or direct left atrial pressure trace (Figure 3.58). In severe aortic regurgitation, the aortic diastolic pressure may equalize with the left ventricular end-diastolic pressure and demands early surgical intervention (Figure 3.59). However, there is a risk of systemic embolization if contact is made with loose or friable vegetations when attempting to obtain coronary arteriograms (Figure 3.60) and crossing potentially infected aortic valves should be avoided [71].

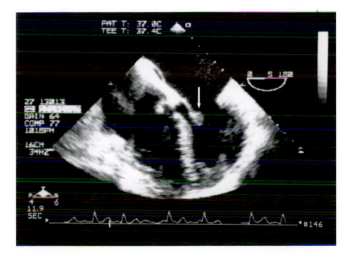

FIGURE 3.34 Transesophageal echocardiogram (TEE) showing large mobile vegetation on mitral valve (arrow) in a diabetic patient with *Streptococcus sanguis* infective endocarditis.

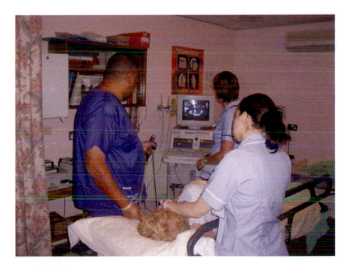

FIGURE 3.36 The cardiologist can maneuver the TEE probe using both hands, so that all views of relevant intracardiac anatomy can be obtained.

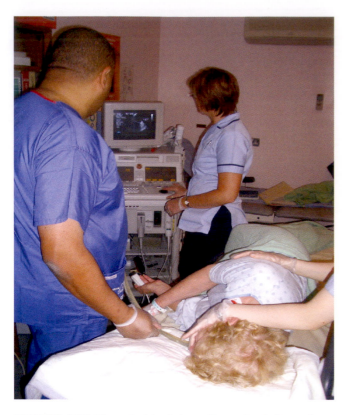

FIGURE 3.37 The technician/echocardiographer helps to focus in on areas of interest, record Doppler color flow images as well as monitor the patient's arterial oxygen saturation using pulse oximetry.

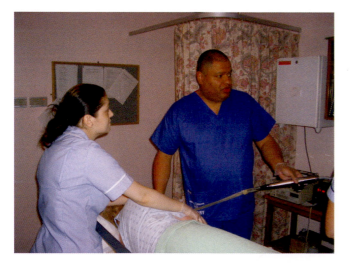

FIGURE 3.38 The proximal end of the TEE probe has controls for angulating the transducer tip in the relevant direction.

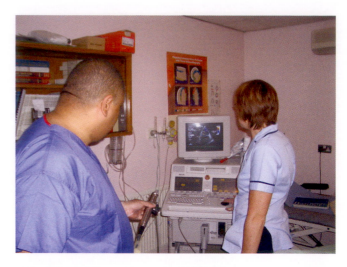

FIGURE 3.39 Images are stored digitally on a modern ECHO machine.

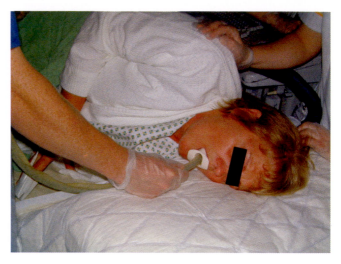

FIGURE 3.40 The TEE probe is protected by a sheath and placed through a mouthpiece to protect the probe from damage by teeth.

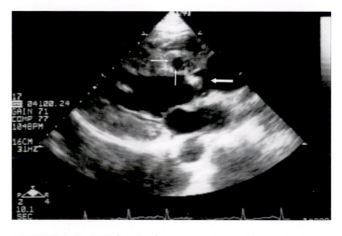

FIGURE 3.41 TEE showing large vegetation on bioprosthetic aortic valve (arrow) infected by coagulase-negative *Staphylococcus*. A large paravalvular abscess is clearly visible (twin arrows).

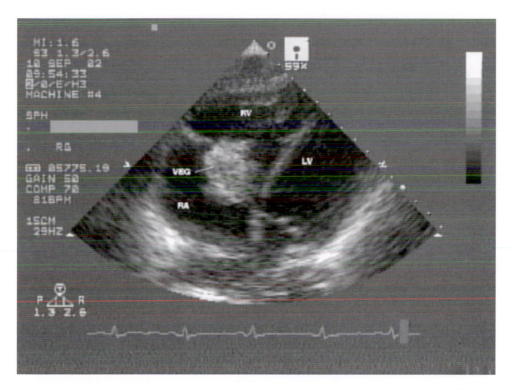

FIGURE 3.42 A 2-D echocardiogram showing large (4 cm diameter) vegetation (VEG) on the tricuspid valve in an IV drug abuser. RV, right ventricle; LV, left ventricle; RA, right atrium. Courtesy of Dr Brad Munt and Dr Rob Moss. Heart 2003;89:577–581. Reproduced with permission from the BMJ Publishing Group.

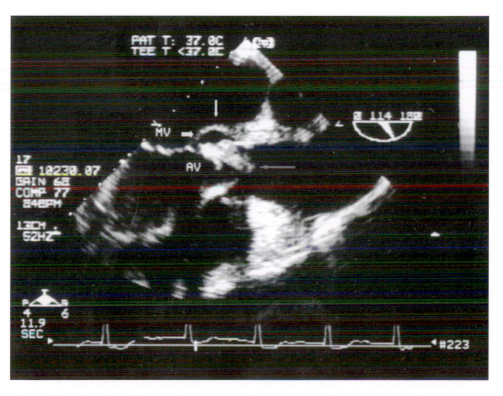

FIGURE 3.43 A 2-D transthoracic echocardiogram showing vegetation on a bioprosthetic aortic valve (single gray arrow) and aortic-root abscess (double white arrows) in a patient with *Staphylococcus epidermidis* endocarditis.

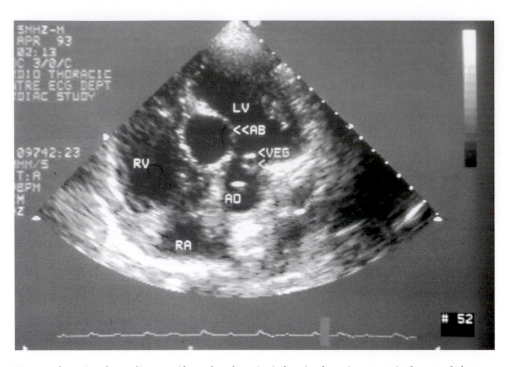

FIGURE 3.44 A 2-D transthoracic echocardiogram (four-chamber view) showing large interventricular septal abscess as a result of *Staphylococcus aureus* infective endocarditis of the aortic valve. This serious complication may result in conduction disturbances such as complete heart block. LV, left ventricle; RV, right ventricle; Ao, aorta; RA, right atrium; <<AB, septal abscess; <<VEG, vegetation. Courtesy of Dr Lindsay Morrison.

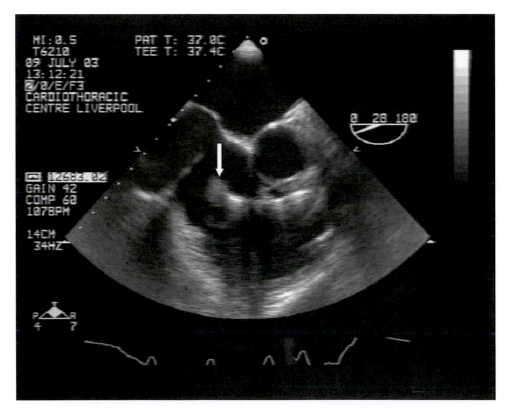

FIGURE 3.45 TEE in a patient with pyrexia 3 months after AICD implantation. A large globular vegetation (arrow) is seen attached to the ventricular lead on the atrial side of the tricuspid valve. It was associated with moderate tricuspid regurgitation due to *Staphylococcus aureus* endocarditis affecting the tricuspid valve. Courtesy of Dr M. Burgess.

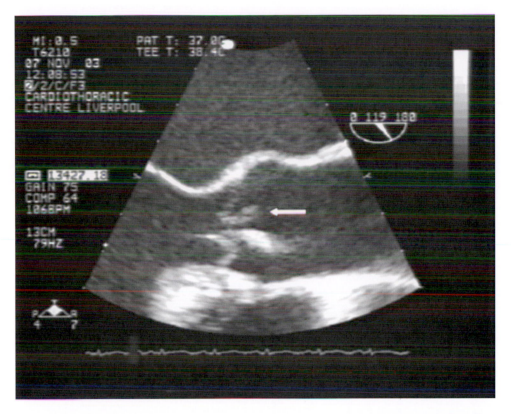

FIGURE 3.46 TEE showing a large vegetation on the noncoronary cusp of the aortic valve (arrow) in an IV drug abuser with severe aortic regurgitation. The vegetation was prolapsing into the left ventricular outflow tract in diastole. Courtesy of Dr M. Burgess.

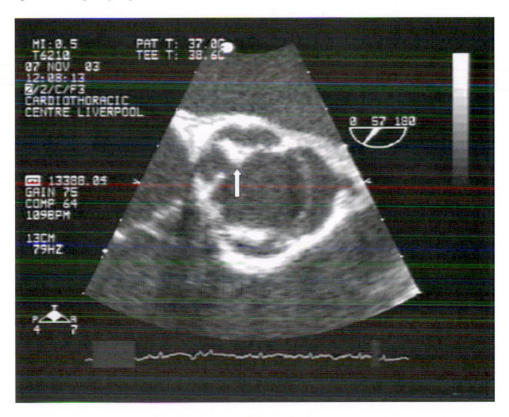

FIGURE 3.47 Same case as in Figure 3.46; TEE. Parasternal short axis view shows vegetation (arrow) on aortic valve leaflet.

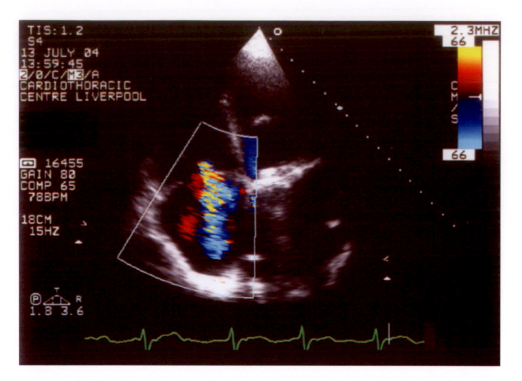

FIGURE 3.48 Color flow transthoracic echocardiogram showing severe tricuspid regurgitation into right atrium.

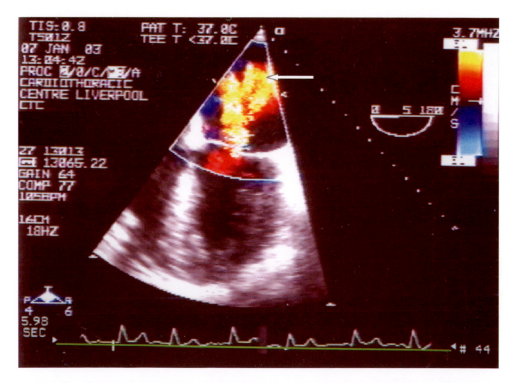

FIGURE 3.49 Color flow TEE shows severe mitral regurgitation (arrow) across a mitral valve infected by *Streptococcus sanguis*.

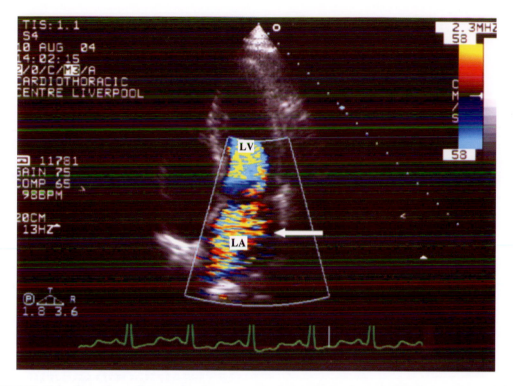

FIGURE 3.50 Color flow echocardiogram showing severe mitral regurgitation (arrow). LV, left ventricle; LA, left atrium.

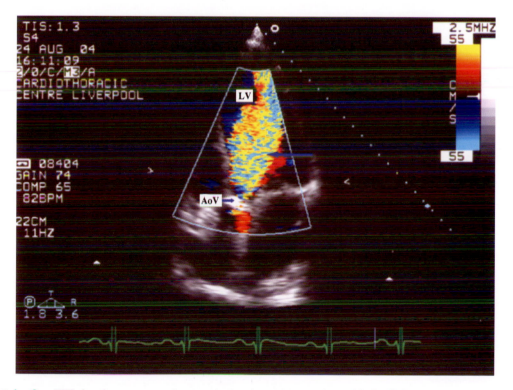

FIGURE 3.51 Color flow TEE showing severe aortic regurgitation (arrow) in a patient with *Staphylococcus aureus* infective endocarditis of the aortic valve. Apical four-chamber view. LV, left ventricle; AoV, aortic valve.

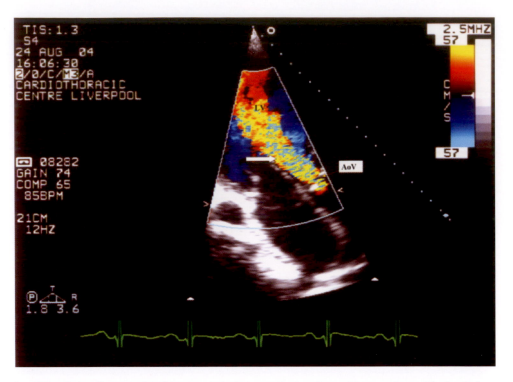

FIGURE 3.52 Color flow echocardiogram showing severe aortic regurgitation (arrow) in a patient with *Staphylococcus aureus* infective endocarditis of the aortic valve. LV, left ventricle; AoV, aortic valve.

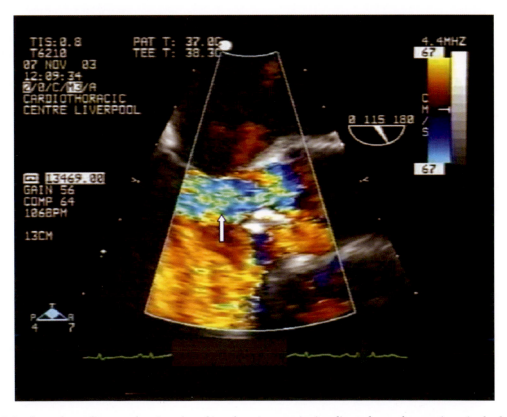

FIGURE 3.53 Color flow echocardiogram showing a broad jet of aortic regurgitation directed onto the anterior mitral valve leaflet—a result of infective endocarditis due to *Coxiella burnetii*.

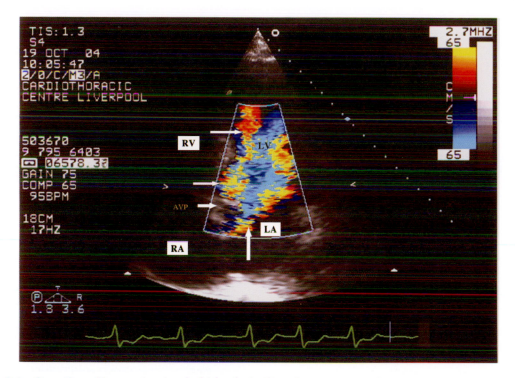

FIGURE 3.54 Color flow echocardiogram showing the high velocity flow of severe paraprosthetic aortic regurgitation (green arrows) and aorta to left atrial fistula (blue arrow) in a 75-year-old man with *Staphylococcus aureus* infective endocarditis of a prosthetic aortic valve (AVP). An aortic root abscess was associated with the severe paraprosthetic aortic regurgitation and a fistulous communication between aorta and left atrium (LA). There was also a vegetation on the atrial aspect of the mitral valve. LV, left ventricle; RA, right atrium; RV, right ventricle.

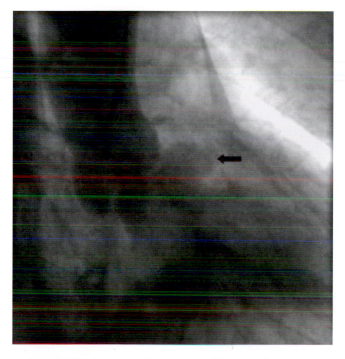

FIGURE 3.55 Aortogram in a 70-year-old man with infective endocarditis of the aortic valve due to viridans streptococci. The illustration shows severe aortic regurgitation and an aneurysm of the sinus of Valsalva (arrow).

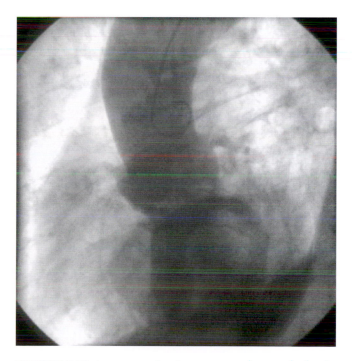

FIGURE 3.56 Aortogram showing severe aortic regurgitation in a man with infective endocarditis of the aortic valve.

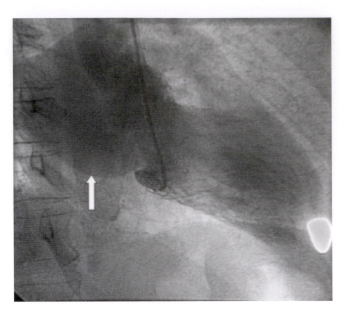

FIGURE 3.57 Left ventricular angiogram showing severe mitral regurgitation into the left atrium (arrow) in a patient with infective endocarditis of the mitral valve.

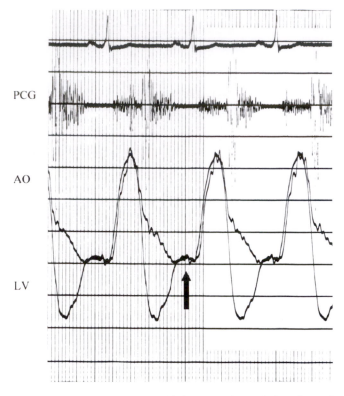

FIGURE 3.59 Equalization of left ventricular end-diastolic and aortic diastolic pressures (arrow) in severe aortic regurgitation due to aortic valve cusp perforation and dehiscence caused by *Staphylococcus aureus* infective endocarditis.

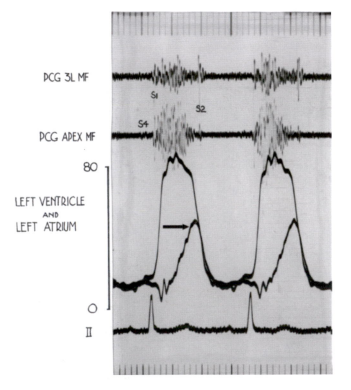

FIGURE 3.58 Phonocardiogram (PCG) shows the pansystolic murmur of mitral regurgitation associated with infective endocarditis of the mitral valve. The intracardiac pressure tracing shows the tall "V" wave (arrow) recorded in the left atrium due to severe mitral regurgitation. (MF = mid-frequency)

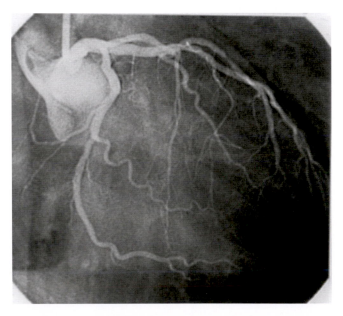

FIGURE 3.60 Coronary arteriography may be indicated to define the presence and extent of coronary artery disease in patients with a history of angina pectoris or myocardial infarction or who possess multiple coronary risk factors but also require surgical intervention for their infective endocarditis.

REFERENCES

1. McCartney AC, Orange GV, Pringle SD, et al. Serum C reactive protein in infective endocarditis. J Clin Pathol 1988;41:44–48.
2. Hogevik H, Olaison L, Andersson R, Alestig K. C-reactive protein is more sensitive than erythrocyte sedimentation rate for diagnosis of infective endocarditis. Infection 1997;25:82–85.
3. Olaison L, Hogevik H, Alestig K. Fever, C-reactive protein, and other acute-phase reactants during treatment of infective endocarditis. Arch Intern Med 1997;157:885–892.
4. Lamas CC, Eykyn SJ. Suggested modifications to the Duke criteria for the clinical diagnosis of native valve and prosthetic valve endocarditis: analysis of 118 pathologically proven cases. Clin Infect Dis 1997;25:713–719.
5. Powers DL, Mandell GL. Intraleukocytic bacteria in endocarditis patients. JAMA 1974;227:312–313.
6. Williams RC. Rheumatoid factors in subacute bacterial endocarditis and other infectious diseases. Scand J Rheumatol Suppl 1988;75:300–308.
7. Asherson RA, Tikly M, Staub H, et al. Infective endocarditis, rheumatoid factor and cardiolipin antibodies. Ann Rheum Dis 1990;49:107–108.
8. Durack D, Lukes A, Bright D. The Duke Endocarditis Service. New criteria for diagnosis of infective endocarditis: utilization of specific echocardiographic findings. Am J Med 1994;96:200–209.
9. Roberts NK, Somerville J. Pathological significance of electrocardiographic changes in aortic valve endocarditis. Br Heart J 1969;31:395–396.
10. Wang K, Gobel F, Gleason DF, et al. Complete heart block complicating endocarditis. Circulation 1972;46:939–947.
11. Arnett EN,, Roberts WC. Valve ring abscess in active infective endocarditis. Circulation 1976;54:140–145.
12. Berk WA. Electrocardiographic findings in infective endocarditis. J Emerg Med 1988;6:129–132.
13. Roggenkamp A, Leitritz L, Baus K, Falsen E, Heesemann J. PCR for detection and identification of *Abiotrophia* spp. J Clin Microbiol 1998;36:2844–2846.
14. Goldenberger D, Kunzli A, Vogt P, Zbinden R, Altwegg M. Molecular diagnosis of bacterial endocarditis by broad-range PCR amplification and direct sequencing. J Clin Microbiol 1997;35:2733–2739.
15. Qin X, Urdahl KB. PCR and sequencing of independent genetic targets for the diagnosis of culture negative bacterial endocarditis. Diagn Microbiol Infect Dis 2001;40:145–149.
16. Wilck MB, Wu Y, Howe JG, et al. Endocarditis caused by culture-negative organisms visible by Brown and Brenn staining: utility of PCR and DNA sequencing for diagnosis. J Clin Microbiol 2001;39:2025–2027.
17. Watkin RW, Lang S, Lambert PA, Littler WA, Elliott TSJ. The microbial diagnosis of infective endocarditis. J Infect 2003;47:1–11.
18. Washington JA II. The role of the microbiology laboratory in the diagnosis and antimicrobial treatment of infective endocarditis. Mayo Clin Proc 1982;57:22–32.
19. Washington JA II. The microbiological diagnosis of infective endocarditis. J Antimicrob Chemother 1987;20:29–39.
20. Werner AS, Cobbs CG, Kaye D, Hook EW. Studies on the bacteremia of bacterial endocarditis. JAMA 1967;202:199–203.
21. Weinstein M, Reller L, Murphy J, Lichenstein K. Clinical significance of positive blood cultures: a comprehensive analysis of 500 episodes of bacteraemia and fungemia in adults. I. Laboratory and epidemiologic observations. Rev Infect Dis 1983;5:35–53.
22. Belli J, Waisbren BA. The number of blood cultures necessary to diagnose most cases of bacterial endocarditis. Am J Med Sci 1956;232:284–288.
23. Weinstein M, Reller L, Murphy J, Lichenstein K. Clinical significance of positive blood cultures: a comprehensive analysis of 500 episodes of bacteraemia and fungemia in adults. I. Clinical observations, with special reference to factors influencing prognosis. Rev Infect Dis 1983;5:54–70.
24. Barnes PD, Crook DWM. Culture negative endocarditis. J Infect 1997;35:209–213.
25. Pesanti EL, Smith IM. Infective endocarditis with negative blood cultures. An analysis of 52 cases. Am J Med 1979;66:43–50.
26. Van Scoy RE. Culture-negative endocarditis. Mayo Clin Proc 1982;57:149–154.
27. Pazin GJ, Saul S, Thompson ME. Blood culture positivity: suppression by outpatient antibiotic therapy in patients with bacterial endocarditis. Arch Intern Med 1982;142;263–268.
28. Hoen B, Selton-Suty C, Lacassin F, et al. Infective endocarditis in patients with negative blood cultures: analysis of 88 cases from a one-year nationwide survey in France. Clin Infect Dis 1995;20:501–506.
29. Mallen MS, Hube EL, Brenes M. Comparative study of blood cultures made from artery, vein and bone marrow in patients with subacute bacterial endocarditis. Am Heart J 1947;33:692–695.
30. Geraci JE, Wilson WR. Endocarditis due to gram-negative bacteria: report of 56 cases. Mayo Clin Proc 1982;57:145–148.
31. Chen YC, Chang SC, Luh KT, Hsieh WC. *Actinobacillus actinomycetemcomitans* endocarditis: a report of four cases and review of literature. Q J Med 1992;81:871–878.
32. Drancourt M, Birtles R, Chaumentin G, et al. New serotype of *Bartonella henselae* in endocarditis and cat-scratch disease. Lancet 1996;347:441–443.
33. Doern GV, Davaro R, George M, Campognone G, et al. Lack of requirement for prolonged incubation of Septi-Chek blood culture bottles in patients with bacteremia due to fastidious bacteria. Diagn Microbiol Infect Dis 1996;24:141–143.
34. Raoult D, Fournier PE, Drancourt M, et al. Diagnosis of 22 new cases of *Bartonella* endocarditis. Ann Intern Med 1996;125:646–652.
35. Editorial. Vegetations, valves and echocardiography. Lancet 1988;ii:1118–1119.

36. Buda AJ, Zotz RJ, Le Mire MS, Bach DS. Prognostic significance of vegetations detected by two-dimensional echocardiography in infective endocarditis. Am Heart J 1986;112:1291–1296.

37. Erbel R, Rohmann S, Drexler M, et al. Improved diagnostic value of echocardiography in patients with infective endocarditis by transoesophageal approach. A prospective study. Eur Heart J 1988;9:43–53.

38. Mugge A, Daniel WG, Franck G, Lichtlen PR. Echocardiography in infective endocarditis: reassessment of prognostic implications of vegetation size determined by the transthoracic and the transesophageal approach. J Am Coll Cardiol 1989;14:631–638.

39. Schwinger ME, Tunick PA, Freedberg RS, Kronzon I. Vegetations on endocardial surfaces struck by regurgitant jets: Diagnosis by transesophageal echocardiography. Am Heart J 1990;119:1212–1215.

40. Taams MA, Gussenhoven EJ, Bos E, et al. Enhanced morphological diagnosis in infective endocarditis by transoesophageal echocardiography. Br Heart J 1990;63:109–113.

41. Steckelberg JM, Murphy JG, Ballard D, et al. Emboli in infective endocarditis: the prognostic value of echocardiography. Ann Intern Med 1991;114:635–640.

42. Birmingham GD, Rahko PS, Ballantyne F 3rd, et al. Improved detection of infective endocarditis with transesophageal echocardiography. Am Heart J 1992;123:774–781.

43. Gilbert BW, Haney RS, Crawford F, et al. Two-dimensional echocardiographic assessment of vegetative endocarditis. Circulation 1977;55:346–353.

44. Plehn JF. The evolving role of echocardiography in management of bacterial endocarditis. Chest 1988;94:904–906.

45. Stewart JA, Silimperi D, Harris P, et al. Echocardiographic documentation of vegetative lesions in infective endocarditis: clinical implications. Circulation 1980;61:374–380.

46. Irani WN, Grayburn PA, Alfredi I. A negative transthoracic echocardiogram obviates the need for transesophageal echocardiography in patients with suspected native valve active infective endocarditis. Am J Cardiol 1996;78:101–103.

47. Klodas E, Edwards WD, Khandheria BK. Use of transesophageal echocardiography for improving detection of valvular vegetations in subacute bacterial endocarditis. J Am Soc Echocardiogr 1989;2:386–389.

48. Nihoyannopoulos P, Oakley CM, Exadactylos N, et al. Duration of symptoms and the effects of a more aggressive surgical policy: two factors affecting prognosis of infective endocarditis. Eur Heart J 1985;6:380–390.

49. Kupferwasser LI, Darius H, Muller AM, et al. Diagnosis of culture-negative endocarditis: the role of the Duke criteria and the impact of transesophageal echocardiography. Am Heart J 2001;142:146–152.

50. Tingleff J, Egeblad H, Gotzsche CO, et al. Perivalvular cavities in endocarditis: abscesses versus pseudoaneurysms? A transesophageal Doppler echocardiographic study in 118 patients with endocarditis. Am Heart J 1995;130:93–100.

51. Tunick PA, Freedberg RS, Schrem SS, Kronzon I. Unusual mitral annular vegetation diagnosed by transesophageal echocardiography. Am Heart J 1990;120:444–446.

52. Jaffe WM, Morgan DE, Pearlman AS, Otto CM. Infective endocarditis. 1983–1988: echocardiographic findings and factors influencing morbidity and mortality. J Am Coll Cardiol 1990;15:1227–1233.

53. Martin RP. The diagnostic and prognostic role of cardiovascular ultrasound in endocarditis: bigger is not better. J Am Coll Cardiol 1990;15:1234–1237.

54. Rohmann S, Erbel R, Gorge G, et al. Clinical relevance of vegetation localization by transoesophageal echocardiography in infective endocarditis. Eur Heart J 1992;12:446–452.

55. Shapiro SM, Bayer AS. Transesophageal and Doppler echocardiography in the diagnosis and management of infective endocarditis. Chest 1991;100:1125–1130.

56. Pedersen WR, Walker M, Olson JD, et al. Value of transesophageal echocardiography as an adjunct to transthoracic echocardiography in evaluation of native and prosthetic valve endocarditis. Chest 1991;100:351–356.

57. Daniel W, Mugge A, Martin R, et al. Improvement in the diagnosis of abscesses associated with endocarditis by transesophageal echocardiography. N Engl J Med 1991;324:795–800.

58. Job FP, Gronke S, Lethen H, et al. Incremental value of biplane and multiplane transesophageal echocardiography for the assessment of active infective endocarditis. Am J Cardiol 1995;75:1033–1037.

59. Lowry RW, Zoghbi WA, Baker WB, et al. Clinical impact of transesophageal echocardiography in the diagnosis and management of infective endocarditis. Am J Cardiol 1994;73:1089–1091.

60. Culver DL, Cacchione J, Stern D, et al. Diagnosis of infective endocarditis on a Starr-Edwards prosthesis by transesophageal echocardiography. Am Heart J 1990;119:972–973.

61. Shapiro S, Young E, De Guzman S, et al. Transesophageal echocardiography in diagnosis of infective endocarditis. Chest 1994;105:377–382.

62. Leung D, Cranney G, Hopkins A, Walsh W. Role of transesophageal echocardiography in the diagnosis and management of aortic root abscess. Br Heart J 1994;72:175–181.

63. Rohmann S, Erbel R, Mohr-Kahaly S, Meyer J. Use of transoesophageal echocardiography in the diagnosis of abscess in infective endocarditis. Eur Heart J 1995;16(Suppl B):54–62.

64. Vered Z, Mossinson D, Peleg E, et al. Echocardiographic Assessment of prosthetic valve endocarditis. Eur Heart J 1995;16(Suppl B):63–67.

65. Mukhtari O, Horton CJ Jr, Nanda NC, et al. Transesophageal color Doppler three-dimensional echocardiographic detection of prosthetic aortic valve dehiscence: correlation with surgical findings. Echocardiography 2001;18:393–397.

66. Martin RP, French JW, Popp RL. Clinical utility of two-dimensional echocardiography in patients with bioprosthetic valves. Adv Cardiol 1980;27:294–304.

67. Shapiro S, Kupferwasser LI. Echocardiography predicts embolic events in infective endocarditis. J Am Coll Cardiol 2001;37:1077–1079.

68. Di Salvo G, Habib G, Pergola V, et al. Echocardiography predicts embolic events in infective endocarditis. J Am Coll Cardiol 2001;37:1069–1076.

69. Heinle S, Wilderman N, Harrison JK, et al. Value of transthoracic echocardiography in predicting embolic events in active endocarditis. Duke Endocarditis Service. Am J Cardiol 1994;74:799–801.

70. Evangelista A, Gonzalez-Alujas MT. Echocardiography in infective endocarditis. Heart 2004;90:614–617.

71. Ward C. Cardiac catheterisation in patients with infective endocarditis. J R Coll Physicians Lond 1997;31:341–342.

CHAPTER 4

Diagnostic Criteria

DUKE CRITERIA FOR DIAGNOSIS OF INFECTIVE ENDOCARDITIS

Criteria for the diagnosis of IE were proposed by von Reyn and colleagues in 1981 based on analysis of symptoms, clinical signs, and blood cultures [1]. These were subsequently refined by Durack and colleagues at the Duke Endocarditis Service in 1994, taking into account information obtained by echocardiography and introducing the concept of major and minor diagnostic criteria [2] (Table 4.1). The advantages and limitations of the Duke criteria for the diagnosis of IE have been studied and modified but echocardiographic data, serology, and culture of excised tissue appear to improve the specificity and sensitivity of the diagnostic criteria [3–17]. Comparison has also been made between the Duke and other criteria (Beth Israel) for the diagnosis of IE and although the modified Duke criteria appear to be superior, confirmatory studies are few and small [18,19]. Larger studies are needed.

More recently, it has been proposed that PCR amplification of specific gene targets and universal loci for bacteria and fungi and subsequent sequencing to identify the possible causative organisms in blood culture and excised tissue should be considered as a major Duke criterion [20]. Such molecular methods have been validated in the diagnosis of CNE and recently implemented into the newest revision of the Duke criteria [21,22].

Diagnosis of "definite" IE requires the presence of two major or one major plus three minor criteria or five minor criteria and has a specificity of around 99% and sensitivity of >80% [2,23].

Histological Techniques

A variety of specialized stains and immunohistological techniques (immunoperoxidase staining, enzyme-linked immunosorbent (ELISA) and immunofluorescent (ELIFA) assays, and direct immunofluorescence using fluorescein conjugated monoclonal antibodies) are now available to allow the identification of elusive bacteria and fungi.

Tissue stains include acridine orange and Giemsa for any bacteria, tissue Gram stain for Gram-positive/negative bacteria, periodic acid–Schiff for *Tropheryma whipplei* and fungi, Gimenez for *Coxiella burnetii* and *Legionella* species, and the Grocott–Gomori stain for fungi [24,25].

Molecular Techniques

The polymerase chain reaction (PCR) utilizing nucleic acid target or signal amplification, alone or in combination with sequence analysis, is most widely used and allows quick and reliable detection of fastidious and difficult-to-culture organisms in blood and tissue removed from patients with infective endocarditis [21] (Figures 4.1–4.3).

16S rRNA genes are found in all bacteria. "Broad-range" or "universal" PCR primers are available to identify "conserved" bacterial 16S rRNA gene sequences and used to amplify intervening, variable, or diagnostic regions. Both 16S (bacterial) rRNA and 18S/28S rRNA (fungal) amplification should be followed by automated sequence identification of the amplicons. "Specific" primers are available for organisms such as *T. whipplei*, *C. burnetii*, *Bartonella*, *Chlamydia*, *Brucella*, *Legionella*, *Mycobacterium*, and *Mycoplasma* species (Figure 4.4).

TABLE 4.1 Duke Criteria for Diagnosis of Infective Endocarditis and Terminology Used in the Modified Diagnostic Criteria

Definite infective endocarditis
Pathological criteria
    Microorganisms: demonstrated by culture or histology in a vegetation that has embolized, or in an intracardiac
      abscess, or
    Pathological lesions: vegetation or intracardiac abscess present, confirmed by histology showing active
      endocarditis
Clinical criteria (use definitions below)
    2 major criteria, or
    1 major and 3 minor criteria, or
    5 minor criteria

Possible infective endocarditis
Findings consistent with IE that fall short of "definite", but not "rejected"

Rejected
Firm alternate diagnosis for manifestations of endocarditis, or
Resolution of manifestations of endocarditis, with antibiotic therapy for 4 days or less, or
No pathological evidence of IE at surgery or autopsy, after antibiotic therapy for 4 days or less

DEFINITIONS

Major criteria
1. Positive blood culture for IE
    Isolation of microorganism known to cause IE from two separate blood cultures, e.g. viridans streptococci, *S. bovis, S. aureus,*
    S. epidermidis, enterococci, *Haemophilus* spp., *Actinobacillus* spp. etc.
    Persistently positive blood culture—defined as recovery of a microorganism consistent with endocarditis from:
    (i) at least two blood cultures drawn more than 12 hours apart, or
    (ii) all of three or a majority of four or more separate blood cultures, with first and last drawn at least
      1 hour apart
2. Evidence of endocardial involvement
    Positive echocardiogram for IE:
    (i) mobile intracardiac mass on valve or supporting structures or in path of
      regurgitant jet, or on implanted material without any alternative anatomical explanation, or
    (ii) abscess, or
    (iii) new partial dehiscence of prosthetic valve, or new valve regurgitation
3. Clinical evidence of new valvular regurgitation
4. Positive serology for Q-fever or other causes of culture-negative endocarditis such as *Bartonella* spp. and
    Chlamydia psittaci
5. Positive identification of a microorganism from blood culture or excised tissue using molecular
    biology methods

Minor criteria
Predisposition: predisposing heart condition or IV drug abuse
Fever: >38.0°C
Vascular phenomena: major arterial emboli, septic pulmonary infarcts, mycotic aneurysm, intracranial
    hemorrhage, conjunctival hemorrhages, Janeway lesions, *newly diagnosed clubbing, splinter hemorrhages, splenomegaly*[a]
Immunological phenomena: glomerulonephritis, Osler's nodes, Roth spots, +ve rheumatoid factor, *high*
    ESR (> 1.5 times upper limit of normal), high C-reactive protein level (> 100 mg/L)[a]
Microbiological evidence: positive blood culture, but not meeting major criteria as defined above

[a] Additional modifications to the Duke criteria appear to improve diagnostic sensitivity whilst retaining specificity.

Collection of clinical specimen
(Blood, blood culture, valve, vegetation, embolic tissue)

↓

DNA extraction

↓

PCR amplification
(Universal/broad-range bacteria 16S, 16-23S, 23S rDNA
Universal/broad-range fungi 18S, 28S, ITS1, ITS2 rDNA
Specific gene target)

↓

Detection of amplicons
(Agarose gel electrophoresis, fluorescence detection-light cycler)

↓

Direct automated DNA sequencing

↓

Bioinformatics/Sequence analysis
(BLAST, FASTA)

FIGURE 4.1 Molecular biology techniques, in particular the polymerase chain reaction (PCR), have allowed for an increased ability to detect and identify causal organisms associated with infective endocarditis. As molecular techniques are rapidly evolving, several permutations exist both in approach and techniques employed. Like all other molecular diagnostic assays, employment of detection and identification schemes for cardiac and cardiovascular specimens follows the general workflow of (1) obtaining such specimens, (2) extraction of microbial DNA, (3) amplification of target gene loci, and (4) identification of amplicon. Courtesy of Dr B. Cherie Millar and Dr John E. Moore.

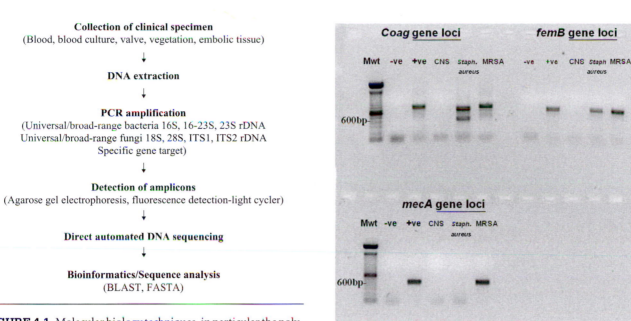

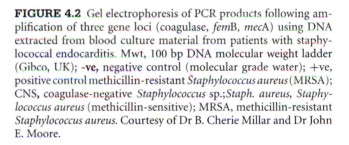

FIGURE 4.2 Gel electrophoresis of PCR products following amplification of three gene loci (coagulase, *femB*, *mecA*) using DNA extracted from blood culture material from patients with staphylococcal endocarditis. Mwt, 100 bp DNA molecular weight ladder (Gibco, UK); **-ve,** negative control (molecular grade water); +ve, positive control methicillin-resistant *Staphylococcus aureus* (MRSA); CNS, coagulase-negative *Staphylococcus* sp.; *Staph. aureus, Staphylococcus aureus* (methicillin-sensitive); MRSA, methicillin-resistant *Staphylococcus aureus*. Courtesy of Dr B. Cherie Millar and Dr John E. Moore.

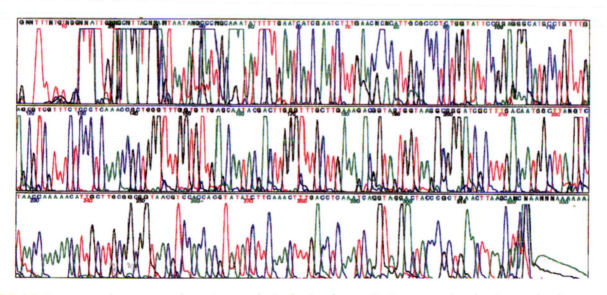

FIGURE 4.3 A representative sequence chromatogram obtained using dye termination sequencing chemistry and a direct automated sequencer (Model 373A, Applied Biosystems, Foster City CA, USA). In this chromatogram, approximately 320 bases have been called from raw unprocessed sequence data of ribosomal RNA gene loci of *Candida albicans*. Courtesy of Dr B. Cherie Millar and Dr John E. Moore.

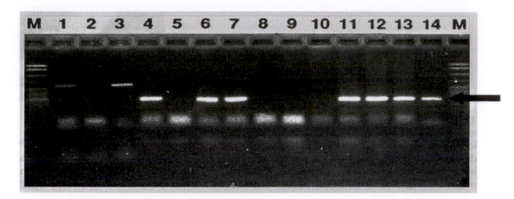

FIGURE 4.4 Polymerase chain reaction (PCR) and DNA amplification techniques can detect DNA from microorganisms that are present in too few numbers to be visualized or when growth characteristics are such that there would be a delay in diagnosis. Advantages of the technique are speed, automation, high degree of specificity and sensitivity, crude extract is satisfactory, and the inoculum need not be viable. The amplified DNA products can then be visualized by agarose gel electrophoresis and staining of DNA with ethidium bromide, which intercalates between the nucleotide bases and fluoresces under ultraviolet light. Here fragments of the expected size (bp) of DNA from *T. whipplei* are identified (arrow) by agarose gel electrophoresis. This organism may cause severe spondylodiskitis and infective endocarditis. Courtesy of Professor M. Altwegg.

Possible quantification by real-time PCR may eliminate the need for gel electrophoresis, with faster, more accurate results and the possibility of investigating common antimicrobial-resistance genes enabling a targeted approach to antibiotic treatment [26].

REFERENCES

1. von Reyn C, Levy B, Arbeit R, Friedland G, Crumpacker C. Infective endocarditis: an analysis based on strict case definitions. Ann Intern Med 1981;94:505–518.
2. Durack D, Lukes A, Bright D. The Duke Endocarditis Service. New criteria for diagnosis of infective endocarditis: utilization of specific echocardiographic findings. Am J Med 1994;96:200–209.
3. Heiro M, Nikoskelainen J, Hartiala JJ, et al. Diagnosis of infective endocarditis. Sensitivity of the Duke vs von Reyn criteria. Arch Intern Med 1998;158:18–24.
4. Habib G, Derumeaux G, Avierinos JF, et al. Value and limitations of the Duke criteria for the diagnosis of infective endocarditis. J Am Coll Cardiol 1999;33:2023–2029.
5. Hoen B, Beguinot I, Raboud C, et al. The Duke criteria for diagnosing infective endocarditis are specific: analysis of 100 patients with acute fever or fever of unknown origin. Clin Infect Dis 1996;23:298–302.
6. Cecchi E, Parrini I, Chinaglia A, et al. New diagnostic criteria for infective endocarditis. A study of sensitivity and specificity. Eur Heart J 1997;18:1149–1156.
7. Olaison L, Hogevik H. Comparison of the von Reyn and Duke criteria for the diagnosis of infective endocarditis: a critical analysis of 161 episodes. Scand J Infect Dis 1996;28:399–406.
8. Dodds GA, Sexton DJ, Durack DT, et al. Negative predictive value of the Duke criteria for infective endocarditis. Am J Cardiol 1996;77:403–407.
9. Muhlestein JB. Infective endocarditis: how well are we managing our patients? J Am Coll Cardiol 1999;33:794–795.
10. Delahaye F, Rial MO, de Gevigney G, et al. A critical appraisal of the quality of the management of infective endocarditis. J Am Coll Cardiol 1999;33:788–793.
11. Rognon R, Kehtari R. Individual value of each of the Duke criteria for the diagnosis of infective endocarditis. Clin Microbiol Infect 1999;5:396–403.
12. Fournier PE, Casalta JP, Habib G, et al. Modification of the diagnostic criteria proposed by the Duke Endocarditis Service to permit improved diagnosis of Q fever endocarditis. Am J Med 1996;100:629–633.
13. Lamas CC, Eykyn SJ. Suggested modification to the Duke criteria for the clinical diagnosis of native valve and prosthetic valve endocarditis: analysis of 118 pathologically proven cases. Clin Infect Dis 1997;25:713–719.
14. Lamas CC, Eykyn SJ. Blood culture negative endocarditis: analysis of 63 cases presenting over 25 years. Heart 2003;89:258–262.
15. Shapiro S, Kupferwasser LI. Echocardiography predicts embolic events in infective endocarditis. J Am Coll Cardiol 2001;37:1077–1079.
16. Di Salvo G, Habib G, Pergola V, et al. Echocardiography predicts embolic events in infective endocarditis. J Am Coll Cardiol 2001;37:1069–1076.
17. Heinle S, Wilderman N, Harrison JK, et al. Value of transthoracic echocardiography in predicting embolic events in active endocarditis. Duke Endocarditis Service. Am J Cardiol 1994;74:799–801.

18. Hoen B, Selton-Suty C, Danchin N, et al. Evaluation of the Duke criteria versus the Beth Israel criteria for the diagnosis of infective endocarditis. Clin Infect Dis 1995;21:905–909.

19. Naber CK, Bartel T, Eggebrecht H, et al. Diagnosis of endocarditis today: Duke criteria or clinical judgement? Herz 2001;26:379–390.

20. Millar BC, Moore JE, Mallon P, et al. Molecular diagnosis of infective endocarditis—a new Duke's criterion. Scand J Infect Dis 2001;33:673–680.

21. Grijalva M, Horvath R, Dendis M, et al. Molecular diagnosis of culture-negative infective endocarditis: clinical validation in a group of surgically treated patients. Heart 2003;89:263–268.

22. Lisby G, Gutschik E, Durack DT. Molecular methods for diagnosis of infective endocarditis. Infect Dis Clin North Am 2002;16:393–412.

23. Li JS, Sexton DJ, Mick N, et al. Proposed modifications to the Duke's criteria for the diagnosis of infective endocarditis. Clin Infect Dis 2000;30:633–638.

24. Lepidi H, Durack DT, Raoult D. Diagnostic methods. Current best practices and guidelines for histologic evaluation in infective endocarditis. Infect Dis Clin North Am 2002;16:339–361.

25. Houpikian P, Raoult D. Diagnostic methods. Current best practices and guidelines for identification of difficult-to-culture pathogens in infective endocarditis. Infect Dis Clin North Am 2002;16:377–392.

26. Moore JE, Millar BC, Yongmin X, et al. A rapid molecular assay for the detection of antibiotic resistance determinants in cause of infective endocarditis. J Appl Microbiol 2001;90:719–726.

CHAPTER 5

Treatment: Prophylaxis

TREATMENT

Despite medical treatment, IE continues to cause significant morbidity and mortality (20%). Prevention therefore is a priority as is early diagnosis and adequate management based on appropriate antibiotic therapy and in many cases cardiac surgery. Antimicrobial prophylaxis before selected procedures in patients at risk has become routine in most countries, despite the fact that no prospective study has been performed that proves that such therapy is definitely beneficial [1–3]. Animal experiments and some human studies have, however, suggested benefit from prophylactic antibiotics [4]. Even if prophylaxis is effective, it can only prevent a minority of cases of endocarditis and it is not cost-effective as a general strategy. Nevertheless, current "best practice" continues to favor the use of antibiotic prophylaxis of selected patients at risk of IE who are undergoing procedures that can cause bacteremia. Guidelines and advice have been published by expert groups in both Europe and the USA and the differences in recommendations are minor [5–10]. However, the guidelines represent consensus recommendations based mainly on data from animal models, case-control studies and case series.

PROPHYLAXIS

In view of these issues, it is prudent to classify the risk of subgroups of patients with preexisting cardiac disorders for developing IE as high, moderate or low, especially since certain cardiac conditions are associated with endocarditis more often than others and the severity of the disease and the resulting morbidity is more severe [8]. Although concerns have been expressed about the value of antibiotic prophylaxis [3,11–19], the fact that animal experiments and clinical experience document IE following bacteremia, that bacteremia occurs after various dental and instrumental procedures, and that antibiotics are available that can kill potential causative organisms, it is prudent to offer prophylactic antibiotic therapy to individuals who are at higher risk of IE than the general population [20–29]. It is particularly important for those in whom IE is associated with high morbidity and mortality [4,5,8,30,31].

It is important to inform those at risk and provide them with written instructions [32]. Although the British Heart Foundation "Endocarditis Dental Warning Card" should currently be given to all patients at risk of developing IE (Figure 5.1), an improvement would be a card that indicates the patient's details, diagnosis, the estimated risk category, whether there is allergy to penicillin, and who to contact for advice about the need for antibiotic prophylaxis if any medical or dental practitioner is contemplating any invasive procedure likely to cause bacteremia. Patients should be told to show the card to their doctor or dentist and there should be written communication between these professionals [33].

Cardiac conditions may be stratified into high-, moderate-, and low-risk groups based on potential outcome if IE should develop.

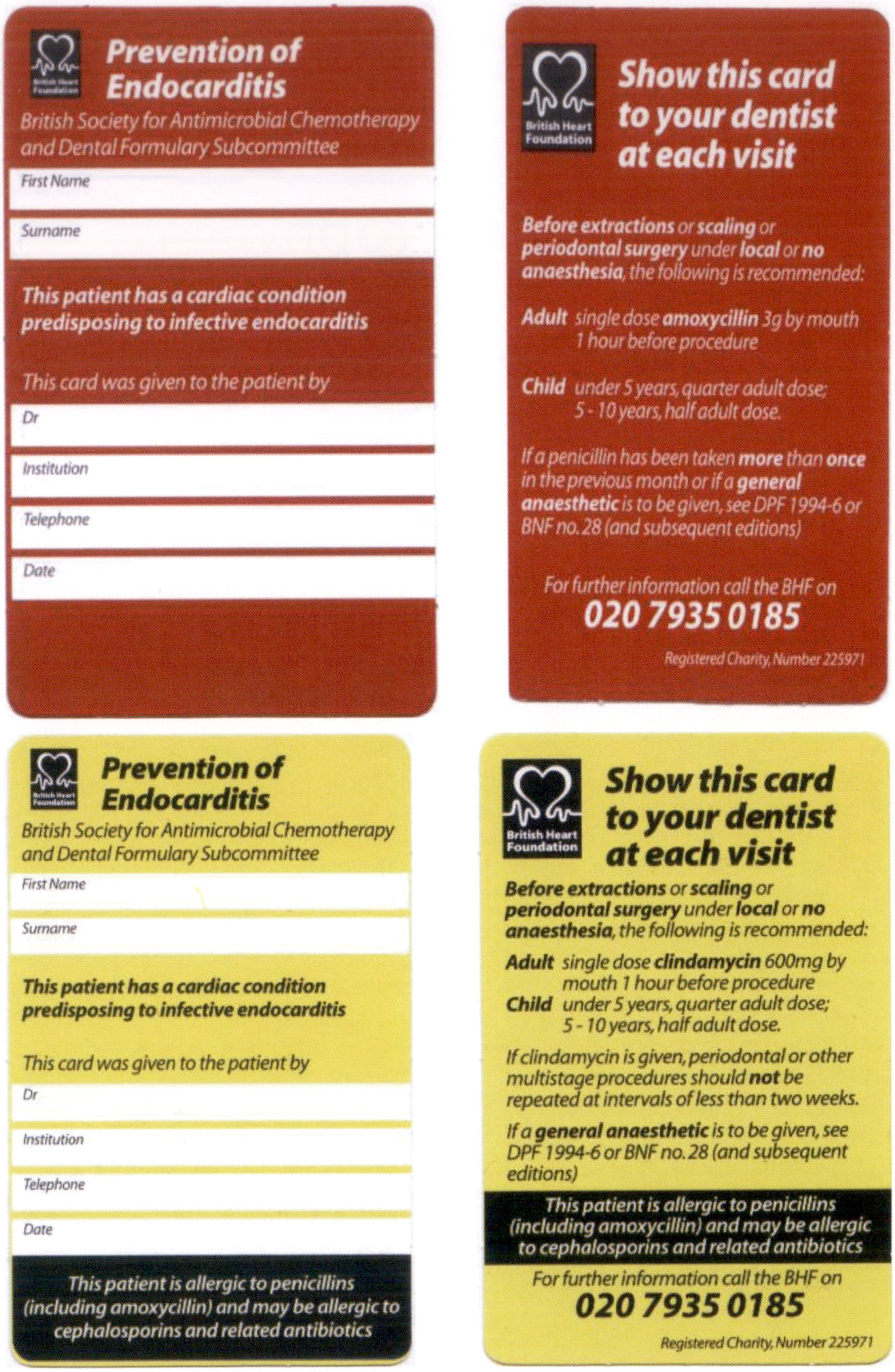

FIGURE 5.1 British Heart Foundation "Endocarditis Dental Warning Cards" for patients requiring dental prophylaxis with antibiotics. The red card should be given to patients who may receive penicillin and the yellow card to those allergic to penicillin.

TABLE 5.1 Antibiotic prophylaxis for high-, moderate-, and low-risk cases

High risk
Previous infective endocarditis [34]
Complex cyanotic congenital heart disease, transposition of great arteries, Fallot's tetralogy, Gerbode's defect [35–37]
Surgically constructed systemic pulmonary shunts or conduits
Mitral valve prolapse with mitral regurgitation or thickened valve leaflets [38–42]
Prosthetic heart valves (5 times greater than those with native valves) [43,44]

Moderate risk
Acquired valvular heart disease, e.g. rheumatic heart disease—aortic stenosis, aortic regurgitation, mitral regurgitation
Non-cyanotic congenital cardiac defects, e.g. bicuspid aortic valve, primum atrial septal defect, patent ductus arteriosus [45], coarctation of
 aorta [47], atrial septal aneurysm/patent foramen ovale [48], ventricular septal defect [49]
Other structural cardiac defects, e.g. aortic root replacement [46], hypertrophic obstructive cardiomyopathy [50–53],subaortic membrane
 [54]

Low-risk cases not requiring antibiotic prophylaxis
Isolated secundum atrial septal defect[a] [55], pulmonary stenosis
Surgically-repaired atrial septal defect, ventricular septal defect or patent ductus arteriosus, post Fontan or Mustard procedure without
 residual defect/murmur
Previous coronary artery bypass surgery
Mitral valve prolapse without regurgitation
Innocent heart murmurs[b]
Cardiac pacemakers/defibrillators[c,d]
Coronary artery stent implantation[c]
Heart/Heart and lung transplant[e]

[a] Antibiotic prophylaxis is recommended for up to 12 months after ASD/PFO catheter-based closure procedures.
[b] If unsure as to the exact nature of the murmur and the need for prophylaxis, an opinion should be sought from a cardiologist. In an emergency or when it is difficult to obtain specific advice then antibiotic prophylaxis should be given prior to dental or surgical treatment.
[c] Unless being performed in patients at moderate or high risk of endocarditis, when antibiotic prophylaxis is advisable.
[d] Pre- and post-procedure antibiotics are generally used routinely for surgical prophylaxis.
[e] Within the first 6 months after heart/heart-lung transplantation, patients should receive antibiotic prophylaxis.

Patients at Risk

Subgroups of patients with preexisting cardiac disorders may be classified at high, moderate, or low risk of developing IE in the event of significant bacteremia occurring following an interventional procedure. Table 5.1 stratifies these cardiac conditions into risk groups based on the outcome should IE develop and the increased susceptibility to IE compared with those in the general population.

Patients at highest risk are those who have prosthetic heart valves, a history of previous endocarditis, complex cyanotic congenital heart disease, surgically constructed systemic pulmonary shunts or conduits. Mitral valve prolapse with mitral regurgitation or thickened leaflets should also be considered in this risk category. Those with prosthetic valves are 5–10 times more at risk than those with native valve disease [34–44].

Congenital cardiac conditions at moderate risk of endocarditis include primum atrial septal defect, ventricular septal defect, patent ductus arteriosus, bicuspid aortic valve and coarctation of the aorta. Patients with rheumatic valve disease or hypertrophic obstructive cardiomyopathy should also be considered at moderate risk [45–55].

Low-risk patients are those patients with cardiac disease in whom the risk is no higher than in the general population and include some patients with grown-up congenital heart (GUCH) disease [36]. Those with innocent heart murmurs and structurally normal hearts do not require antibiotic prophylaxis.

Procedures Requiring Antibiotic Prophylaxis

Bacteremia commonly occurs during chewing and toothbrushing [56–58]. However, significant bacteremia causing IE seems to occur most often after certain procedures. These procedures include dental procedures and instrumentation of the oral/respiratory, gastrointestinal, or genitourinary tracts [59–64]. The evidence for many other procedures is limited [4,65–74].

The risk of developing IE is probably directly related to the frequency and severity of bacteremia that occurs with each individual procedure and its duration, and the procedure/portal of entry is a determinant of the organism involved and the type of prophylaxis regimen that should be appropriate [75,76]. What constitutes a "significant" degree of bacteremia has been a matter of much debate and research, and in the area of dentistry, the work has proved helpful in defining which procedures are associated with the greatest yield of bacteremia and hence especially worthy of antibiotic prophylaxis [77–79]. For

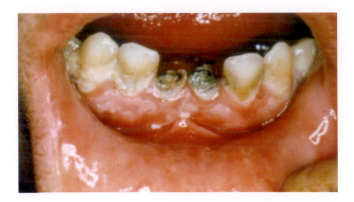

FIGURE 5.2 Severe dental caries and gingivitis in a patient with infective endocarditis of the mitral valve due to *Streptococcus mitis*. Transient bacteremia occurs with dental extraction and periodontal surgery, but also spontaneously in the presence of severe periodontal disease. Courtesy of Mr Phil Hardy.

example, bleeding after dental treatment is not in itself associated with an increased frequency of bacteremia and this has changed advice about antibiotic prophylaxis for certain dental procedures.

DENTAL AND ORAL PROCEDURES

Poor dental hygiene and periodontal or periapical infections may produce bacteremia even in the absence of dental procedures and so those at risk of endocarditis should establish and maintain the best possible oral hygiene to minimize the risk [61,80,81] (Figures 5.2 and 5.3). This can be aided by regular dental follow-up and

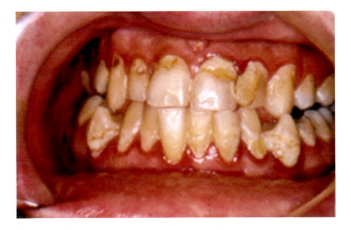

FIGURE 5.3 Severe dental caries resulting in *Streptococcus sanguis* infective endocarditis of both mitral and aortic valves. Courtesy of Mr Phil Hardy.

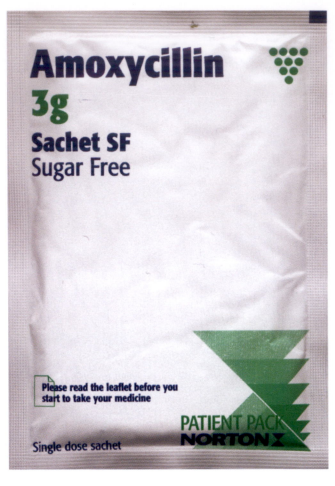

FIGURE 5.4 A 3 g sachet of amoxicillin is used as prophylaxis against IE in those patients at risk of developing endocarditis who are undergoing dental procedures.

care and daily techniques to minimize plaque build-up, e.g. toothbrushing, dental floss, plaque removal. However, even these simple procedures may not be without risk [82,83]. Chlorhexidine mouthwash (0.2%), preferably non-alcoholic, may help patients who find a high standard of plaque control difficult. Although recent work has questioned its effectiveness, 15 ml of chlorhexidine hydrochloride (0.2%) should be given as an oral rinse to all patients at risk 5 minutes prior to dental treatment to reduce the incidence and magnitude of odontogenic bacteremia [80,84–86]. Sustained or repeated frequent interval use is not indicated as this may result in the selection of resistant organisms.

Antibiotic prophylaxis for at-risk patients is recommended for dental and oral procedures likely to cause bacteremia [61,62,87,88] (Figure 5.4). The dental procedures that require prophylaxis are shown in Table 5.2.

TABLE 5.2 Dental procedures and endocarditis antibiotic prophylaxis for high- and moderate-risk cases [115,116]

Prophylaxis required	Prophylaxis not required
Examination procedures Periodontal probing [117]	Dental examination with mirror and probe [79]
Investigative procedures Sialography [118]	Intraoral radiographs Extraoral radiographs
Preventive procedures Nil	Fissure sealants Fluoride treatments
Professional cleaning procedures[a] Polishing teeth with a rubber cup [119,120] Air polishing [121] Oral irrigation with water jet [122,123] Light scaling [124,125] Deep scaling [124,125] Scaling teeth with hand instrument [120,126] Scaling with ultrasonic instrument [126]	
Anesthetic procedures Intraligamental local anesthetic injections [99]	Infiltration local anesthetic injections [99] Nerve block local anesthesia Oral airway for GA [127,128] Nasal airway for GA [127–129] Laryngeal mask airway for GA [130,131]
Comprehensive dental treatment under general anesthesia [132] Extractions and fillings [133–135]	
Conservative (restorative) procedures[b] Rubber dam placement [136,137] Matrix band and wedge placement [136,137] Gingival retraction cord placement [137]	Slow and fast drilling of teeth (without rubber dam) [136,137]
Periodontal procedures Root planing (similar to scaling) Antibiotic fibers or strips placed subgingivally[c] Gingivectomy [124] Periodontal surgery [138]	
Endodontic procedures[d] Root canal instrumentation beyond the apex [124,139] Avulsed tooth reimplantation[e] Non-vital pulpotomy of primary molar	Root canal instrumentation within the root canal [139] Vital pulpotomy of primary molar [140,141] Pulpotomy of permanent tooth [f]
Orthodontic procedures [142,143] Tooth separation [77] Expose or expose and bond tooth/teeth [143]	Alginate impressions [77] Placement of removable appliances Band placement and cementation [77,91,144] Band removal [92] Adjustment of fixed appliances [77,145]
Surgical procedures Extraction of single tooth [124,132,143,146,147] Extraction of multiple teeth [124,143,146,149] Incision and drainage of an abscess with extraction Mucoperiosteal flap to gain access to tooth or lesion [143,150] Dental implants (as for mucoperiosteal flap)	Incision and drainage of an abscess without extraction [148] Dental implants—transmucosal fixture
Post-surgical procedures	Suture removal [131–133] Removal of surgical packs
Daily or physiological events	Exfoliation of primary teeth Toothbrushing Flossing Use of interdental wooden points

[a] There is a paradox inherent in endocarditis prophylaxis in that many cleaning procedures, i.e. toothbrushing, dental flossing, interdental wooden points, oral irrigation all cause a significant bacteremia. There is no justification for using antibiotic prophylaxis for these self-care procedures carried out at home on a daily or twice daily basis.

[b] It is common for a course of dental treatment to take several visits to the dentist. For patients at high or moderate risk of developing infective endocarditis, as much treatment as possible should be carried out at each visit. The antibiotic should be changed at alternate visits, e.g. amoxicillin—clindamycin—amoxicillin etc., but no more than two doses of penicillin should be given within a month. For patients who are allergic to penicillin, then a period of 1 month must be allowed between visits.

[c] No data but the procedure is very similar to gingival retraction cord placement.

[d] Dental treatment confined to the root canal does not require antibiotic prophylaxis. However, if a rubber dam is used, antibiotic prophylaxis should be used since significant bacteremia often results in these circumstances.

[e] The avulsed tooth can be quickly washed and reimplanted immediately and the antibiotic prophylaxis administered when the child attends the dental surgery provided this is within 2 hours of the reimplantation. This is because antibiotic prophylaxis is still successful if administered after the bacteremic episode [98].

[f] No data but the procedure is similar to pulpotomy of primary molar.

Prophylaxis against IE in orthodontics has been discussed in the literature [77,89,90]. However, this is a specially difficult problem as some procedures cause significant bacteremia (e.g. tooth separation) but others such as banding and debanding cause only a small, nonsignificant increase in bacteremia [88,91,92]. It is possible that the deterioration in gingival health as a consequence of the appliances placed in the mouth is a risk factor that needs to be considered more carefully. If patients are unable to maintain good oral hygiene when appliances are in the mouth, it may be helpful to use a chlorhexidine mouthwash for the period of the appliance therapy [93,94].

Antibiotics administered up to 1 hour before a dental procedure will effect a reduction in odontogenic bacteremia and a most important clinical advance was the demonstration that oral administration of amoxicillin proved effective in significantly reducing dental bacteremia [95]. This has become the mainstay of outpatient dental care both in general and in specialist practice. Regimens for IV or IM administration have also been tested and proved to be effective for adults and children [96,97].

Data from experimental animal models suggest that antimicrobial prophylaxis administered within 2 hours following the procedure will also provide protection [98]. However, antibiotics given >4 hours after the procedure probably have no prophylactic benefit. Intraligamental injections of local anaesthetic should be avoided if possible as severe bacteremia occurs in a large proportion of patients [99].

For patients undergoing cardiac surgery, a careful preoperative dental evaluation is recommended so that necessary dental treatment can be completed before cardiac surgery whenever possible in an attempt to reduce the incidence of late postoperative IE.

OTHER PROCEDURES

Antibiotic prophylaxis is recommended in patients at high or moderate risk of IE who are undergoing various gastrointestinal, genitourinary, respiratory, or cardiac procedures and subspecialty societies have published their guidelines for antibiotic prophylaxis [100–103]. These procedures are listed in Table 5.3. The evidence for significant bacteremia after many of theses procedures has not been proven, but since cases of infective endocarditis have been reported to follow them, prophylactic antibiotics are recommended (Figs 5.5 and 5.6). Some procedures do not require antibiotic prophylaxis.

TABLE 5.3 Other procedures requiring endocarditis prophylaxis in high-and moderate-risk cases

Prophylaxis required
Gastrointestinal tract
　Esophageal procedures [154,155]
　Surgical operations on stomach, small or large bowel
　Endoscopic retrograde cholangiography/biliary obstruction [156]
　Endoscopy with/without biopsy [100–102,157–161]
　Endoscopic variceal sclerotherapy [161,162]
　Percutaneous endoscopic gastrostomy [103]
　Biliary tract surgery
　Lithotripsy of gallstones [163]
Genitourinary tract
　Circumcision [164]
　Prostatic surgery, transrectal biopsy [165]
　Vasectomy [166,167]
　Lithotripsy [168]
　Cystoscopy
　Urethral catheterization in presence of bacteriuria
　Urethral dilatation
　Gynecological operations, e.g. hysterectomy, cesarean section, vaginal delivery[a] [169,170]
　Therapeutic abortion [171–173], uterine dilatation and curettage, sterilization procedures, insertion of intrauterine device[a] [174]
　Removal of infected intrauterine devices[a]
　Smears[a] [175]
Respiratory tract
　Tonsillectomy/adenoidectomy
　Surgical procedures on respiratory tract
　Bronchoscopy—particularly rigid bronchoscopy [176,177]
　Nasal packing[a] [178]
Cardiac
　Implantation of cardiac pacemakers/defibrillators [179–181]
　Cardiac surgical operations
　Implantation of occlusive devices, e.g. ductal occluders [182], septal occluders [183,184]
　Transesophageal echocardiography[a] [185]
　Balloon valvuloplasty [186–190]
　Balloon dilatation of coarctation of aorta[a] [191]
　PTCA/PCI/Stent implantation[a] [192,193]
Ophthalmological
　Lacrimal duct probing[a] [194]
Dermatological
　Surgery[a] [195,196]
Other
　Thermal injury/burns[a] [197,198]
　Acupuncture[a] [199,200]
　Body piercing[a] [201–203]
　Tattooing[a] [204]
Prophylaxis not required
Gastrointestinal tract—barium examinations
Genitourinary tract—urethral catheterization—unless bacteriuria evident
Respiratory tract—endotracheal intubation
Cardiac—diagnostic cardiac catheterization

[a] Although not considered "high-risk" procedures, bacteremia and/or IE have been reported after these procedures and antibiotic prophylaxis should be considered for those patients considered at high or moderate risk of IE (Table 5.2). The ESC did not recognize these to be indications for antibiotic prophylaxis in their Task Force Report [10,205].

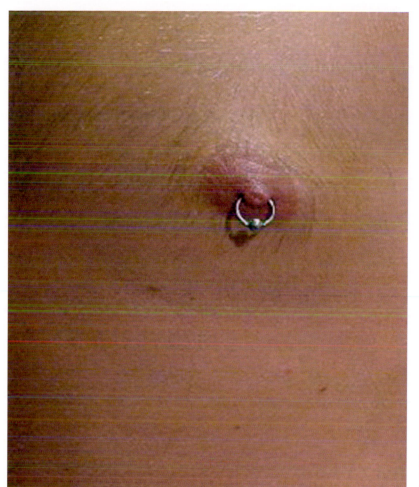

FIGURE 5.5 Body piercing may be associated with infective endocarditis in patients at risk because of their cardiac lesion.

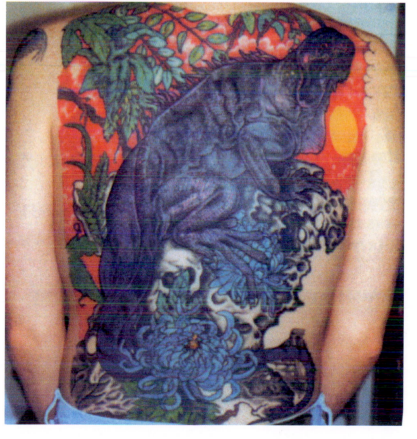

FIGURE 5.6 Tattooing may involve driving up to 14 dye-impregnated needles into the dermis several hundred times per minute. In persons at increased risk of infective endocarditis such as those with prosthetic valves, staphylococcal bacteraemia may result in infective endocarditis. Patients should be advised against such body decoration or at least offered antibiotic prophylaxis prior to the procedure. Courtesy of Dr. Peter Schofield and colleagues and reproduced with permission from the BMJ Publishing Group. Heart 2001;85:11–12.

TABLE 5.4 Prophylactic antibiotic regimens for dental, oral, respiratory tract, or esophageal procedures in adults

Clinical situation	Drug	Regimen
High-risk and moderate-risk patients including those with prosthetic valves[a]	Amoxicillin	3 g oral 1 h pre-procedure or 2 g IV <30 min pre-procedure[b]
For those patients allergic to penicillin[c]	Clindamycin[d] [206]	600 mg oral/300 mg IV 1 h/<30 min pre-procedure[e] then oral or IV clindamycin 150 mg 6 hours later
	or azithromycin[d]	500 mg oral 1 h pre-procedure
	or vancomycin +gentamicin	1 g IV over 2 hours, 1–2 h pre-procedure 1.5 mg/kg IV <30 min pre-procedure[b]
	or teicoplanin +gentamicin	400 mg IV <30 min pre-procedure[b] 1.5 mg/kg <30 min pre-procedure[b]
Patients with previous infective endocarditis[f]	Amoxicillin +gentamicin	2 g IV 1 h pre-procedure + 1 g IV/orally at 6 h 1.5 mg/kg IV <30 min pre-procedure[b]
For those patients allergic to penicillin[c]	Vancomycin +gentamicin	1 g IV over 2 h, 1–2 h pre-procedure 1.5 mg/kg IV <30 min pre-procedure[b]

[a] Particular care should be taken to ensure that patients with prosthetic heart valves are protected by prophylactic antibiotics, since the consequences of infective endocarditis are particularly serious. It is essential that they receive prophylactic antibiotics at least 1 hour before the procedure. If not, they should be given IV antibiotics immediately before the procedure or the procedure should be postponed.
[b] For those undergoing GA, IV antibiotics should be given either on induction or within 30 minutes prior to starting the procedure; oral amoxicillin (3 g) should be given 4 hours before induction and again as soon as possible after the procedure. Where oral antibiotics are not ideal and in cases where IV access is difficult or impossible, e.g. IV drug abusers, IM clindamycin 600 mg 1 hour preoperatively or IM teicoplanin (2 mg/kg) 1 hour preoperatively may be alternative treatments.
[c] Or having received a penicillin within the previous 4 weeks.
[d] Azithromycin 500 mg as an oral suspension, given 1 hour before the procedure, may be an alternative if dysphagia is a problem.
[e] Clindamycin to be infused over 10–15 minutes.
[f] These patients are considered to be at particularly high risk of IE.

ANTIBIOTIC PROPHYLAXIS REGIMENS

Antibiotic prophylaxis varies according to the type of procedure being performed and the type of microorganism likely to cause infection. The regimens for prophylaxis for dental, oral, respiratory, or esophageal procedures are shown in Table 5.4 and for genitourinary and gastrointestinal procedures in Table 5.5. A comparison between the regimens used in the UK, Europe, and the USA is shown in Table 5.6. In patients with prosthetic valves, the antibiotics should be given 1 hour before the interventional procedure and 6 hours after the procedure [104,105].

Prior to (and after) permanent pacemaker implantation or cardiac surgery, prophylactic antibiotics are given to prevent serious wound infection, mediastinitis, and endocarditis due to staphylococci, streptococci, and enterococci [106,107]. Institution- or surgeon-specific selection of antibiotics is appropriate [108,109] and some examples of regimens are shown in Tables 5.7 (for pacemaker implantation) and 5.8 (for cardiac surgery). Data suggest that a 1-day course of IV antimicrobials is as efficacious as the traditional 48-hour (or longer) regimens [110–114]. There are insufficient data to suggest that aminoglycosides add substantial benefit to the prophylactic regimen [108].

TABLE 5.5 Prophylactic antibiotic regimens for genitourinary or gastrointestinal procedures in adults

Clinical situation	Drug	Regimen
High-risk and moderate-risk patients	Ampicillin or amoxicillin + gentamicin	2 g IV <30 min pre-procedure[a] and 1 g IV or orally 6 h post-procedure 1.5 mg/kg IV <30 min pre-procedure[a]
For those patients allergic to penicillin	Vancomycin + gentamicin	1 g IV over 2 h, 1–2 h pre-procedure 1.5 mg/kg IV <30 min pre-procedure[a]

[a] For those undergoing GA, the antibiotics should be given either on induction or within 30 minutes prior to starting the procedure.

TABLE 5.6 Antibiotic prophylaxis regimens for high-risk patients: comparison between UK, Europe, and USA

Procedure	UK	Europe	USA
Dental/Oral/Respiratory tract/Esophageal	**Amoxicillin** 2–3 g oral 1 h preop or 2 g IV <30 min preop	**Amoxicillin** 2 g oral 1 h preop or 2 g IV 30–60 min preop **Children:** 50 mg/kg orally/IV 1 h preop	**Amoxicillin** 2 g 1 h preop or 2 g IV/IM <30 min preop **Children:** 50 mg/kg orally 1 h preop
Penicillin allergic	**Clindamycin** 600 mg oral 1 h preop or 300 mg IV <30 min preop then oral or IV Clindamycin 150 mg 6 h post	**Clindamycin** 600 mg oral 1 h preop **Children:** 20 mg/kg orally 1 h preop	**Clindamycin** 600 mg oral 1 h preop or 600 mg IV <30 min preop **Children:** 20 mg/kg orally 1 h preop
Genitourinary/Gastrointestinal	**Ampicillin** 2 g IV <30 min preop **+ gentamicin** 1.5 mg/kg IV <30 min preop **+ ampicillin** 1 G IV or orally 6 hr post	**Ampicillin or amoxicillin** 2 g IV 30–60 min preop **+ gentamicin** 1.5 mg/kg IV <30 min preop **+ ampicillin** 1 G orally 6 hr post **Children:** ampicillin 50 mg/kg IV + gentamicin 1.5 mg/kg 30–60 min preop	**Ampicillin** 2 g IV/IM <30 min preop **+ gentamicin** 1.5 mg/kg <30 min preop **+ ampicillin** 1 G IV/IM or amoxicillin 1 G oral 6 hrs later **Children:** ampicillin 50 mg/kg IM/IV + gentamicin 1.5 mg/kg <30 min preop + ampicillin 25 mg/kg IM/IV or amoxicillin 25 mg/kg orally 6 hrs postop
Penicillin allergic	**Vancomycin** 1 g IV over 2 h, 1–2 h preop **+ gentamicin** 1.5 mg/kg IV <30 min preop	**Vancomycin** 1 g IV over 2 h, 1–2 h preop **+ gentamicin** 1.5 mg/kg IV/IM <30 min preop **Children:** vancomycin 20 mg/kg IV over 1–2 h + gentamicin 1.5 mg/kg IV/IM	**Vancomycin** 1 g IV over 1–2 h <30 min preop **+ gentamicin** 1.5 mg/kg IV/IM <30 min preop **Children:** vancomycin 20 mg/kg IV over 1–2 h + gentamicin 1.5 mg/kg IV/IM

TABLE 5.7 Prophylactic antibiotic regimens for permanent pacemaker implantation[a]

Clinical situation	Drug	Regimen
High-risk and moderate-risk patients	Flucloxacillin[b]	1 g IV <30 min pre-procedure + 500 mg orally four times a day for 2 days
For those patients allergic to penicillin	Vancomycin	1 g IV over 2 h, 1–2 h pre-procedure + erythromycin 500 mg orally four times a day for 2 days

[a] Probably should be followed in high/moderate-risk patients having defibrillator, stent, or other intravascular device implantation.
[b] Patients infected or colonized with MRSA should be given vancomycin rather than flucloxacillin.

TABLE 5.8 Prophylactic antibiotic regimens for cardiac surgery[a]

Procedure	Drug	Regimen
Coronary artery bypass graft surgery	Flucloxacillin 1 g IV	3 doses—first dose given on induction then 8-hourly
	+ gentamicin 1.5 mg/kg IV	3 doses—first dose given on induction then 8-hourly
	or	
	Cefuroxime 1.5 g IV	6 doses—first dose given on induction second after CPB, then 8-hourly
Valvular or other cardiac surgery if any prosthetic device/material is used	Flucloxacillin 1 g IV	3 doses—first dose given on induction then 8-hourly
	+ gentamicin 1.5 mg/kg IV	3 doses—first dose given on induction then 8-hourly
	or	
	Cefuroxime 1.5 g IV	3 doses—first dose given on induction then 8-hourly
	+ vancomycin 1 g IV (infused over 2 h)	3 doses—first dose given on induction then 8-hourly
For those patients allergic to penicillin	Vancomycin 1 g IV (infused over 2 h)	First dose 30–60 min before skin incision, 2 further doses at 12 and 24 h

[a] Prophylactic antibiotics at the time of cardiac surgery are given not only to prevent endocarditis and prosthetic infection but to prevent other serious infections such as mediastinitis and major wound infection [207].
The dose and type of antibiotics varies according to the sensitivity patterns of microorganisms in the cardiac surgical environment and in the individual patient. Some cardiac surgical units use a combination of antibiotics, others use monotherapy.
The timing of antibiotics is important. They should be given prior to surgery and for at least 24–48 hours postoperatively.
In MRSA carriers or in units where there is a high prevalence of infection by MRSA, vancomycin should *always* replace flucloxacillin.

REFERENCES

1. Horstkotte D, Rosin H, Friedrichs W, Loogen F. Contribution for choosing the optimal prophylaxis of bacterial endocarditis. Eur Heart J 1987;8(Suppl J):379–381.

2. Imperpale T, Horwitz T. Does prophylaxis prevent post-dental infective endocarditis? A controlled evaluation of predictive efficacy. Am J Med 1990;88:131–136.

3. van de Meer J, van Wijk W, Thompson J, et al. Efficacy of antibiotic prophylaxis for prevention of native valve endocarditis. Lancet 1992;339:135–139.

4. Durack D. Prevention of infective endocarditis. N Engl J Med 1995;332:38–44.

5. Leport C, Horstkotte D, Burckhardt D and the Group of Experts of the International Society for Chemotherapy. Antibiotic prophylaxis for infective endocarditis from an international group of experts towards a European consensus. Eur Heart J 1995;16(Suppl B):126–131.

6. Advisory Group of the British Cardiac Society Clinical Practice Committee and the Royal College of Physicians Clinical Effectiveness and Evaluation Unit. The Prophylaxis and Treatment of Infective Endocarditis in Adults. www.bcs.com

7. Dajani A, Taubert K, Wilson W, et al. Prevention of bacterial endocarditis. Recommendations by the American Heart Association. Circulation 1997;96:358–366.

8. Simmons NA, Ball AP, Cawson RA, et al. Antibiotic prophylaxis and infective endocarditis. Lancet 1992;339:1292–1293.

9. Simmons NA. Recommendations for endocarditis prophylaxis. The Endocarditis Working Party for Antimicrobial Chemotherapy. J Antimicrob Chemother 1993;31:437–438.

10. The Task Force on Infective Endocarditis of the European Society of Cardiology. Guidelines on Prevention, Diagnosis and Treatment of Infective Endocarditis. Executive Summary. Eur Heart J 2004;25:267–276.

11. Editorial. Chemoprophylaxis for infective endocarditis: faith, hope and charity challenged. Lancet 1992;339:525–526.

12. Seymour RA, Lowry R, Whitworth JM, et al. Infective endocarditis, dentistry and antibiotic prophylaxis; time for a rethink? Br Dent J 2000;189:610–616.

13. Durack DT, Kaplan EL, Bisno AL. Apparent failures of endocarditis prophylaxis. Analysis of 52 cases submitted to a national registry. JAMA 1983;250:2318–2322.

14. Roberts GJ. Dentists are innocent! Everyday bacteraemia is the real culprit: a review and assessment of the evidence that dental surgical procedures are a principal cause of bacterial endocarditis in children. Pediatr Cardiol 1999;20:317–325.

15. Wise R, Hart T, Cars O, et al. Antimicrobial resistance is a major threat to public health. Br Med J 1998;317:609–610.

16. Fleming P, Feigal RJ, Kaplan EL, et al. The development of penicillin-resistant oral streptococci after repeated penicillin prophylaxis. Oral Surgery 1990;70:440–444.

17. Leviner E, Tzukert A, Benoliel R, et al. Development of resistant oral viridans streptococci after administration of prophylactic antibiotics: time management in the dental treatment of patients susceptible to infective endocarditis. Oral Surg Oral Med Oral Pathol 1987;64:417–420.

18. Woodman AJ, Vidic J, Newman HN, Marsh PD. Effects of repeated high dose prophylaxis with amoxycillin on the resident oral flora of adult volunteers. J Med Microbiol 1985;19:15–23.

19. Longman LP, Pearce PK, McGowan P, et al. Antibiotic resistant oral streptococci in dental patients susceptible to infective endocarditis. J Med Microbiol 1991;34:33–37.

20. Lewis T, Grant RT. Observations relating to subacute infective endocarditis. Br Heart J 1923;10:21–77.

21. Taran LM. Rheumatic fever in its relation to dental disease. N Y J Dent 1944;14:107–113.

22. Longman LP, Marsh PD, Martin MV. Amoxycillin resistant oral streptococci and experimental infective endocarditis in the rabbit. J Antimicrob Chemother 1992;30:349–352.

23. Blatter M, Franciolo P. Endocarditis prophylaxis: from experimental models to human recommendation. Eur Heart J 1995;16(Suppl B):107–109.

24. Durack DT, Petersdorf RG. Chemotherapy of experimental streptococcal endocarditis I: Comparison of commonly recommended prophylactic regimens. J Clin Invest 1973;52:592–598.

25. Durack DT, Beeson PB, Petersdorf RG. Experimental bacterial endocarditis III: Production and progress of the disease in rabbits. Br J Exp Pathol 1973;54:142–151.

26. Garrison PK, Freedman LR. Experimental endocarditis I. Staphylococcal endocarditis in rabbits resulting from placement of a polyethylene catheter in the right side of the heart. Yale J Biol Med 1970;42:394–410.

27. Glauser PM, Bernard JP, Morcillon P, Franciolo P. Successful single dose amoxycillin prophylaxis against experimental streptococcal endocarditis: evidence of two mechanisms of protection. J Infect Dis 1983;147:568–575.

28. Malinverni R, Overholsen CD, Bille J, Glauser MP. Antibiotic prophylaxis of experimental endocarditis after dental extraction. Circulation 1988;77:182–187.

29. Strom BL, Abrutyn E, Berlin JA, et al. Dental and cardiac risk factors for infective endocarditis. Ann Intern Med 1998;129:761–769.

30. Strom BL, Abrutyn E, Berlin JA, et al. Risk factors for infective endocarditis: oral hygiene and non-dental exposure. Circulation 2000;102:2842–2848.

31. Delahaye F, De Gevigney G. Should we give antibiotic prophylaxis against infective endocarditis in all cardiac patients, whatever the type of dental treatment? Heart 2001;85:9–10.

32. Cetta F, Warnes CA. Adults with congenital heart disease: patient knowledge of endocarditis prophylaxis. Mayo Clin Proc 1995; 70:50–54.

33. Buckingham JK, Gould IM, Tervitt G, Williams S. Prevention of endocarditis: communication between doctors and dentists. Br Dent J 1992;172:414–415.

34. Lossos IS, Oren R. Recurrent infective endocarditis. Postgrad Med J 1993;69:816–818.

35. Noreuil TO, Katholi RE, Graham DR. Recurrent bacterial endocarditis in a man with tetralogy of Fallot: earliest recurrence on record. South Med J 1990;83:455–457.

36. Li W, Somerville J. Infective endocarditis in the grown-up congenital heart (GUCH) population. Eur Heart J 1998;19:166–173.

37. Michel C, Rabinovitch MA, Huynh T. Gerbode's defect associated with acute sinus node dysfunction as a complication of infective endocarditis. Heart 1996;76:379.

38. Piper C, Horstkotte D, Schulte HD, Schultheib HP. Mitral valve prolapse and infection: a prospective study for risk calculation. Eur Heart J 1996;17(Abstract Suppl):210.

39. Steckelberg JM, Wilson WR. Risk factors for infective endocarditis. Infect Dis Clin North Am 1993;7:9–19.

40. Bisno AL. Mitral valve prolapse and infective endocarditis. Arch Intern Med 1993;153:1506.

41. Carabello BA. Mitral valve disease. Curr Probl Cardiol 1993;7:423–478.

42. Cheng TO. Should antibiotic prophylaxis be recommended for all patients with mitral valve prolapse? Am J Cardiol 1991;68:564.

43. Calderwood SB, Swinski LA, Watermaux CM, et al. Risk factors for the development of prosthetic valve endocarditis. Circulation 1985;72:31–37.

44. Leport C, Vilde JL, Bricaire F, et al. 50 cases of late prosthetic valve endocarditis: improvement in prognosis over a 15 year period. Br Heart J 1987;53:66–71.

45. Mandel KE, Ginsburg CM. Staphylococcal endocarditis complicating a patent ductus arteriosus. Pediatr Infect Dis J 1994;13:833–834.

46. Ralph-Edwards A, David TE, Bos J. Infective endocarditis in patients who had replacement of the aortic root. Ann Thorac Surg 1994;58:429–432.

47. D'Costa DF, Davidson AR. Coarctation of the aorta associated with a sinus venosus atrial septal defect presenting with endocarditis in middle age. Postgrad Med J 1990;66:951–952.

48. Sommer R, Dussoix P, Anwar A, Garbino J. Unusual association: *Streptococcus bovis* tricuspid endocarditis with atrial septal aneurysm and patent foramen ovale. Schweiz Med Wochenschr 2000;130:395–397.

49. Villa E, Mohammedi I, Dupperret S, et al. Community-acquired methicillin-resistant *Staphylococcus aureus* right-sided infective endocarditis in a non-addict patient with ventricular septal defect. Intensive Care Med 1999;25:236–237.

50. Spirito P, Rapezzi C, Bellone P, et al. Infective endocarditis in hypertrophic cardiomyopathy: prevalence, incidence and indications for antibiotic prophylaxis. Circulation 1999;99:2132–2137.

51. Stulz P, Zimmerli W, Mihatsch J, Gradel E. Recurrent infective endocarditis in idiopathic hypertrophic subaortic stenosis. Thorac Cardiovasc Surg 1989;37:99–102.

52. Alessandri N, Pannarale G, del Monte F, et al. Hypertrophic obstructive cardiomyopathy and infective endocarditis: a report of seven cases and a review of the literature. Eur Heart J 1990;11:1041–1048.

53. Chen MR. Infective endocarditis in hypertrophic obstructive cardiomyopathy. J Clin Ultrasound 1992;20:612–614.

54. Pentousis D, Cooper JP, Rae AP. Bacterial endocarditis involving a subaortic membrane. Heart 1996;76:370–371.

55. Rahman A, Burma O, Felek S, Yekeler H. Atrial septal defect presenting with *Brucella* endocarditis. Scand J Infect Dis 2001;33:776–777.

56. Everett ED, Hirschmann JV. Transient bacteremia and endocarditis prophylaxis. A review. Medicine 1977;56:61–77.

57. Cobe HM. Transitory bacteraemia. Oral Surg 1954;7:609–615.

58. Berger SA, Weitzman S, Edberg SC. Bacteraemia after using an oral irrigation device. Ann Intern Med 1974;80:510–511.

59. Meneely JK. Bacterial endocarditis following urethral manipulation. N Engl J Med 1948;239:708–709.

60. Brenman HS, Randall E. Local degerming with povidone-iodine. J Periodontol 1974;45:870–872.

61. Gunteroth WG. How important are dental procedures as a cause of infective endocarditis? Am J Cardiol 1984;130:715–718.

62. Delaye J, Etienne J, Feruglio GA, et al. Prophylaxis of infective endocarditis for dental procedures. Report of a working party of the European Society of Cardiology. Eur Heart J 1985;6:826–828.

63. Slade N. Bacteraemia and septicaemia after urological operations. Proc R Soc Med 1958;51:331–334.

64. Sullivan NM, Sutter VL, Mims MM, et al. Clinical aspects of bacteremia after manipulation of the genitourinary tract. J Infect Dis 1973;127;49–55.

65. Camara DS, Gruber M, Barde CJ, et al. Transient bacteremia following endoscopic injection sclerotherapy of esophageal varices. Arch Intern Med 1983;143:1350–1352.

66. Shorvon PJ, Eykyn SJ, Cotton PB. Gastrointestinal instrumentation, bacteraemia and endocarditis. Gut 1983;24:1078–1093.

67. Edson RS, van Scoy RE, Leary FJ. Gram-negative bacteremia after transrectal needle biopsy of the prostate. Mayo Clin Proc 1980;55:489–491.

68. Livengood CH III, Land MR, Addison WA. Endometrial biopsy, bacteremia and endocarditis risk. Obstet Gynecol 1985;65:678–681.

69. Mellow MH, Lewis RJ. Endoscopy-related bacteremia. Incidence of positive blood cultures after endoscopy of upper gastrointestinal tract. Arch Intern Med 1976;136:667–669.

70. Yin TP, Dellipiani AW. Bacterial endocarditis after Hurst bougienage in a patient with a benign oesophageal stricture. Endoscopy 1983;15:27–28.

71. Giglio JA, Rowland RW, Dalton HP, Laskin DM. Suture removal-induced bacteremia: a possible endocarditis risk. J Am Dent Assoc 1992;123:65–70.

72. Ho H, Zuckerman MJ, Wassem C. A prospective controlled study of the risk of bacteremia in emergency sclerotherapy of esophageal varices. Gastroenterology 1991;101:1642–1648.

73. Low DE, Shoenut JP, Kennedy JK, et al. Prospective assessment of risk of bacteremia with colonoscopy and polypectomy. Dig Dis Sci 1987;32:1239–1243.

74. Biorn CL, Browning WH, Thompson L. Transient bacteremia immediately following transurethral prostatic resection. J Urol 1950;63:155–161.

75. Levison ME, Abrutyn E. Infective endocarditis: current guidelines on prophylaxis. Curr Infect Dis Rep 1999;1:119–125.

76. Lockhart PB. The risk for endocarditis in dental practice. Periodontol 2000;23:127–135.

77. Lucas VS, Omar J, Vieira A, Roberts GJ. The relationship between odontogenic bacteraemia and orthodontic treatment procedures. Eur J Orthodont 2002;24:293–301.

78. Roberts GJ, Gardner P, Simmons NA. Optimum sampling time for detection of odontogenic bacteraemia in children. Int J Cardiol 1992;35:311–315.

79. Roberts GJ, Holzel H, Sury MRJ, et al. Dental bacteraemia in children. Pediatr Cardiol 1997;18:24–27.

80. Okell CC, Elliot SD. Bacteraemia and oral sepsis with special reference to the etiology of subacute endocarditis. Lancet 1935;ii:869–874.

81. Elliot SD. Bacteraemia and oral sepsis. Proc R Soc Med 1939;32:747–754.

82. Jenney AW, Cherry CL, Davis B, Wesselingh SL. "Floss and (nearly) die": dental floss and endocarditis. Med J Aust 2001;174:107–108.

83. Donley TG, Donley KB. Systemic bacteremia following toothbrushing: a protocol for the management of patients susceptible to infective endocarditis. Gen Dent 1988;36:482–484.

84. Pallasch TJ. A critical appraisal of antibiotic prophylaxis. Int Dent J 1989;39:183–196.

85. Bender IB, Naidorf IJ, Garvey GJ. Bacterial endocarditis: A consideration for physician and dentist. J Am Dent Assoc 1984;109:415–420.

86. Lockhart PB. An analysis of bacteremias during dental extractions. Arch Intern Med 1996;156:513–520.

87. Morris AM, Webb GD. Antibiotics before dental procedures for endocarditis prophylaxis: back to the future. Heart 2001;86:3–4.

88. Durack DT. Antibiotics for prevention of endocarditis during dentistry: time to scale back? Ann Intern Med 1998;129:829–831.

89. Samaranayake LP. Orthodontics and infective endocarditis prophylaxis. Br Dent J 1995;179:48.

90. Roberts GJ, Lucas VS, Omar J. Bacterial endocarditis and orthodontics. J R Coll Surg Edinb 2000;45:141–145.

91. Erverdi N, Kadir T, Ozkan H, Acur A. Investigation of bacteraemia after orthodontic banding. Am J Orthod Dentofacial Orthop 1999;116:687–690.

92. Erverdi N, Biren S, Kadir T, Acar A. Investigation of bacteraemia following orthodontic debanding. Angle Orthod 2000;70:11–14.

93. Macfarlane TW, Ferguson MM, Mulgrew CJ. Post-extraction bacteraemia: role of antiseptics and antibiotics. Br Dent J 1984;156:179–181.

94. Stirrups DR, Laws E, Honigan JL. The effect of chlorhexidine gluconate mouthrinse on oral health during fixed appliance orthodontic treatment. Br Dent J 1995;151:84–86.

95. Shanson DC, Ashford RFU, Singh J. High dose oral amoxicillin for preventing endocarditis. Br Med J 1980;280:446–448.

96. Shanson DC, Shehata A, Tadayon M, Harris M. Comparison of intravenous teicoplanin with intramuscular amoxycillin for the prophylaxis of streptococcal bacteraemia in dental patients. J Antimicrob Chemother 1987;20:85–93.

97. Roberts G, Holzel H. Intravenous antibiotic regimens and prophylaxis of odontogenic bacteraemia. Br Dent J 2002;193:525–527.

98. Berney P, Francioli P. Successful prophylaxis of experimental streptococcal endocarditis with single dose amoxicillin administered after bacterial challenge. J Infect Dis 1990;161:281–285.

99. Roberts GJ, Simmons NB, Longhurst PB, Hewitt PB. Bacteraemia following local anaesthetic injections in children. Br Dent J 1998;185:295–298.

100. Mani V, Cartwright K, Dooley J, et al. Antibiotic prophylaxis in gastrointestinal endoscopy: a report by a Working Party for the British Society of Gastroenterology Endoscopy Commmittee. Endoscopy 1997;29:114–119.

101. American Society for Gastrointestinal Endoscopy. Antibiotic prophylaxis for gastrointestinal endoscopy. Gastrointest Endosc 1995;42:630–635.

102. The American Society of Colon and Rectal Surgeons. Practice parameters for antibiotic prophylaxis to prevent infective endocarditis or infected prosthesis during colon and rectal endoscopy. Dis Colon Rectum 1992;35:277.

103. Rey JR, Axon A, Budzynska A, et al. European Society of Gastrointestinal Endoscopy. Guidelines of the European Society of Gastrointestinal Endoscopy (ESGE) antibiotic prophylaxis for gastrointestinal endoscopy. Endoscopy 1998;30:318–324.

104. Hyde JA, Darouiche RO, Costerton JW. Strategies for prophylaxis against prosthetic valve endocarditis: a review article. J Heart Valve Dis 1998;7:316–326.

105. Horstkotte D, Weist K, Ruden H. Better understanding of the pathogenesis of prosthetic valve endocarditis—recent perspectives for prevention strategies. J Heart Valve Dis 1998;7:313–315.

106. Kreter B, Woods M. Antibiotic prophylaxis for cardiothoracic operations: meta-analysis of thirty years of clinical trials. J Thorac Cardiovasc Surg 1992;104:590–599.

107. Townsend TR, Reitz BA, Bilker WB, Bartlett JG. Clinical trial of cefamandole, cefazolin and cefuroxime for antibiotic prophylaxis in cardiac operations. J Thorac Cardiovasc Surg 1993;106:664–670.

108. Eagle KA, Guyton RA, et al. ACC/AHA Guidelines for Coronary Artery Bypass Graft surgery. A Report of the American College of Cardiology/American Heart Association Task Force on Practice Guidelines. J Am Coll Cardiol 1999;34:1262–1347.

109. Ariano RE, Zhanel GG. Antimicrobial prophylaxis in coronary bypass surgery: a critical appraisal. DICP 1999;25:478–484.

110. Vuorisalo S, Pokela R, Syrjala H. Is single-dose antibiotic prophylaxis sufficient for coronary artery bypass surgery? An analysis of peri- and postoperative serum cefuroxime and vancomycin levels. J Hosp Infect 1997;37:237–247.

111. Kriaras I, Michalopoulos A, Michalis A, et al. Antibiotic prophylaxis in cardiac surgery. J Cardiovasc Surg 1997;38:605–610.

112. Kaiser AB, Petracek MR, Lea JW IV, et al. Efficacy of cefazolin, cefamandole and gentamicin as prophylactic agents in cardiac surgery: results of a prospective, randomized, double-blind trial in 1,030 patients. Ann Surg 1987;206:791–797.

113. Niederhauser U, Vogt M, Genoni M, et al. Cardiac surgery in a high risk group of patients: is prolonged postoperative antibiotic prophylaxis effective? J Thorac Cardiovasc Surg 1997;114:162–168.

114. Wellens F, Pirlet M, Larbuisson R, et al. Prophylaxis in cardiac surgery: a controlled randomized comparison between cefazolin and cefuroxime. Eur J Cardiothorac Surg 1995;9:325–329.

115. Simmons NA. Dentistry and endocarditis. Br Dent J 1990;169:74–75.

116. McGowan DA. Dentistry and endocarditis. Br Dent J 1990;169:69.

117. Daly CG, Mitchell DH, Highfield JE, Grossberg DE. Bacteraemia due to periodontal probing: a clinical and microbiological investigation. Periodontol 2001;72:210–214.

118. Lamey PJ, MacFarlane TW, Patton DW, et al. Bacteraemia consequential to sialography. Br Dent J 1985;158:218–220.

119. DeLeo AA, Schoenknecht FD, Anderson MW, Peterson JC. The incidence of bacteraemia following oral prophylaxis on pediatric patients. Oral Surg 1974;37:36–45.

120. Lucas VS, Roberts GJ. Odontogenic bacteremia following tooth cleaning procedures in children. Pediatr Dent 2000;22:96–100.

121. Hunter KM, Holborow DW, Kardos TB, et al. Bacteraemia and tissue damage resulting from air polishing. Br Dent J 1989;167:275–278.

122. Berger SA, Weitzman S, Edberg SC. Bacteraemia after using an oral irrigation device. Ann Intern Med 1974;80:510–511.

123. Felix JE, Rosen S, App GR. Detection of bacteremia after the use of an oral irrigation device in subjects with periodontitis. J Periodontol 1971;42:785–789.

124. Bender IB, Seltzer S, Tashman S, Meloff G. Dental procedures in patients with rheumatic heart disease. Oral Surg Oral Med Oral Pathol 1963;16:466–473.

125. Doerffel W, Fietze I, Baumann G, Witt C. Severe prosthetic valve-related endocarditis following dental scaling: a case report. Quintessence Int 1997;28:271–274.

126. Bandt CL, Korn NA, Schaffer EM. Bacteraemias from ultrasonic and hand instrumentation. J Periodontol 1964;35:214–215.

127. Ali MT, Tremewen DR, Hay AJ, Wilkinson DJ. The occurrence of bacteraemia associated with the use of oral and nasopharyngeal airways. Anaesthesia 1992;47:153–155.

128. Gerber MA, Gastanaduy AS, Buckley J, Kaplan EL. Risk of bacteremia after endotracheal intubation for general anesthesia. South Med J 1987;73:1478–1480.

129. Dinner M, Tjeuw M, Artusio JF. Bacteremia as a complication of nasotracheal intubation. Anesth Analg 1987;66:460–462.

130. Stone JM, Karalliedde LD, Carter ML, Cumerland NS. Bacteraemia and insertion of laryngeal mask airways. Anaesthesia 1992;47:77.

131. Brimacombe J, Shorney N, Swainston R, Bapty G. The incidence of bacteraemia following laryngeal mask insertion. Anaesth Intensive Care 1992;20:484–486.

132. Longman CP, Martin MV. A practical guide to antibiotic prophylaxis in restorative dentistry. Dent Update 1999;26:7–14.

133. Berry FA, Yarbrough S, Yarbrough N, et al. Transient bacteremia during dental manipulation in children. Pediatrics 1973;51:476–479.

134. Roberts GJ, Radford P, Holt R. Prophylaxis of dental bacteraemia with oral amoxycillin in children. Br Dent J 1987;162: 179–182.

135. Kralovic SM, Melin-Aldana H, Smith KK, Linnemann CC Jr. *Staphylococcus lugdunensis* endocarditis after tooth extraction. Clin Infect Dis 1995;20:715–716.

136. Roberts GJ, Gardner P, Longhurst P, Black A, Lucas VS. Intensity of bacteraemia associated with conservative dental procedures in children. Br Dent J 2000;188:95–98.

137. Sonbol H, Spratt D, Roberts GJ, Lucas VS. Bacteraemia from conservative (restorative) procedures. Proceedings of 7th International Symposium on Modern Concepts in Endocarditis; 2002.

138. Lineberger LT, De Marco TJ. Evaluation of transient bacteraemia following routine periodontal procedures. J Periodontol 1973;44:757–763.

139. Debelian GJ, Olsen I, Tronstad L. Bacteremia in conjunction with endodontic therapy. Endod Dent Traumatol 1995;11:142–149.

140. Farrington FH. The incidence of transient bacteremia following pulpotomies on primary teeth. ASDC J Dent Child 1973;40:175–184.

141. Beechen II, Laston DJ, Garbarino VE. Transitory bacteremia as related to the operation of vital pulpotomy. J Oral Surg 1956;9:902–905.

142. Khurana M, Martin MV. Orthodontics and infective endocarditis. Br J Orthod 1999;26:295–298.

143. Roberts GJ, Watts R, Longhurst P, Gardner P. Bacteraemia of dental origin and antimicrobial sensitivity following oral surgical procedures in children. Pediatr Dent 1998;20:28–36.

144. McLaughlin JO, Coulter WA, Coffey A, Burden DJ. The incidence of bacteremia after orthodontic banding. Am J Orthod 1996;109:639–644.

145. Biancaniello TM, Romero JR. Bacterial endocarditis after adjustment of orthodontic appliances. J Pediatr 1991;118:248–249.

146. Peterson LJ, Peacock R. The incidence of bacteremia in pediatric patients following tooth extraction. Circulation 1976;53:676–679.

147. Burket LW, Burn CG. Bacteremias following dental extraction. Demonstration of source of bacteria by means of a non pathogen (*Serratia marcescens*). J Dent Res 1937;16:521–530.

148. Flood TR, Samaranayake LP, Macfarlane TW, et al. Bacteraemia following incision and drainage of dento-alveolar abscesses. Br Dent J 1990;169:51–53.

149. Robinson L, Kraus FW, Lazansky JP, Wheeler RE, Johnson V. Bacteremias of dental origin. II. A study of factors influencing occurrence and detection. Oral Surg Oral Med Oral Pathol 1950;3:923–926.

150. Heimdahl A, Hall G, Hedberg M, et al. Detection and quantitation by lysis-filtration of bacteraemia after different oral surgical procedures. J Clin Microbiol 1990;28:2205–2209.

151. Giglio JA, Rowland RW, Dalton HP, Laskin DM. Suture removal induced bacteremia: a possible endocarditis risk. J Am Dent Assoc 1992;123:69–70.

152. Brown AR, Papasian J, Shultz P, Thiesen D, Shultz RE. Bacteremia and intraoral suture removal: can an antimicrobial rinse help? J Am Dent Assoc 1998;129:1455–1461.

153. King RC, Crawford JJ, Small EW. Bacteraemia following intraoral suture removal. Oral Surg Oral Med Oral Pathol 1988;65:23–28.

154. Zuccaro G Jr, Richter JE, Rice TW, et al. Viridans streptococcal bacteremia after esophageal stricture dilation. Gastrointest Endosc 1998;48:568–573.

155. Meyer GW. Endocarditis prophylaxis for esophageal dilation: a confusing issue? Gastrointest Endosc 1998;48:641–643.

156. Subhani JM, Kibbler C, Dooley JS. Review article: antibiotic prophylaxis for endoscopic retrograde cholangiopancreatography (ERCP). Aliment Pharmacol Ther 1999;73:103–116.

157. Breuer GS, Yinnon AM, Halevy J. Infective endocarditis associated with upper endoscopy: case report and review. J Infect 1998;36:342–344.

158. Norfleet RG. Infectious endocarditis after fiberoptic sigmoidoscopy. With a literature review. J Clin Gastroenterol 1991;13:448–451.

159. Watanakunakorn C. *Streptococcus bovis* endocarditis associated with villous adenoma following colonoscopy. Am Heart J 1988;116:1115–1116.

160. Logan RF, Hastings JG. Bacterial endocarditis: a complication of gastroscopy. Br Med J 1988;296:1107.

161. Baskin G. Prosthetic endocarditis after endoscopic variceal sclerotherapy: a failure of antibiotic prophylaxis. Am J Gastroenterol 1989;84:311–312.

162. Wong A, Rosenstein AH, Rutherford RE, James SP. Bacterial endocarditis following endoscopic variceal sclerotherapy. J Clin Gastroenterol 1997;24:90–91.

163. Kullman E, Jonsson KA, Lindstrom E, et al. Bacteremia associated with extracorporeal shockwave lithotripsy of gallbladder stones. Hepatogastroenterology 1995;42:816–820.

164. Schlesinger Y, Urbach J. Circumcision and endocarditis prophylaxis. Arch Pediatr Adolesc Med 1998;152:412.

165. Roblot F, Le MG, Irani J, et al. Infective endocarditis after transrectal prostatic biopsy. Scand J Infect Dis 2002;34:131.

166. Fervenza FC, Contreras GE, Garratt KN, Steckelberg JM. *Staphylococcus lugdunensis* endocarditis: a complication of vasectomy? Mayo Clin Proc 1999;74:1227–1230.

167. Kessler RB, Kimbrough RC 3rd, Jones SR. Infective endocarditis caused by *Staphylococcus hominis* after vasectomy. Clin Infect Dis 1998;27:216–217.

168. Zimhony O, Goland S, Malnick SD, et al. Enterococcal endocarditis after extracorporeal shock wave lithotripsy for nephrolithiasis. Postgrad Med J 1996;72:51–52.

169. Murai N, Katayama Y, Imazeki T, et al. Post parturition infectious endocarditis in a patient with a normal mitral valve. Jpn J Thorac Cardiovasc Surg 1999;47:171–173.

170. Hughes LO, McFadyen IR, Raftery EB. Acute bacterial endocarditis on a normal aortic valve following vaginal delivery. Int J Cardiol 1988;18:261–262.

171. Pantanovitz L, Hodkinson J, Zeele R, Jones N. Gonococcal endocarditis after threatened abortion: a case report. J Reprod Med 1998;43:1043–1045.

172. Panigrahi NK, Panda RS, Panda S. Tricuspid valve endocarditis following elective abortion. Indian J Chest Dis Allied Sci 1998;40:69–72.

173. Kangavari S, Collins J, Cercek B, et al. Tricuspid valve group B streptococcal endocarditis after an elective termination of pregnancy. Clin Cardiol 2000;23:301–303.

174. Cobbs CG. IUD and endocarditis. Ann Intern Med 1973;78:451.

175. Mong K, Taylor D, Muzyka T, et al. Tricuspid endocarditis following a Papanicolaou smear: case report. Can J Cardiol 1997;13:895–896.

176. Jurado RL, Klein S. Infective endocarditis associated with fiberoptic bronchoscopy in a patient with mitral valve prolapse. Clin Infect Dis 1998;26:768–769.

177. Vigla M, Oren I, Bentur L, et al. Incidence of bacteraemia following fiberoptic bronchoscopy. Eur Respir J 1999;14:789–791.

178. Finelli PF, Ross JW. Endocarditis following nasal packing: need for prophylaxis. Clin Infect Dis 1994;19:984–985.

179. Cacoub P, Leprince P, Nataf P, et al. Pacemaker infective endocarditis. Am J Cardiol 1998;82:480–484.

180. Wagshal AB, Tager S, Maor E, et al. Implantable defibrillator endocarditis. Pacing Clin Electrophysiol 1999;22:1120.

181. Da Costa A, Kirkorian G, Cucherat M, et al. Antibiotic prophylaxis for permanent pacemaker implantation: a meta-analysis. Circulation 1998;97:1796–1801.

182. Latson LA, McManus BM, Doer C, et al. Endocarditis risk of the USCI PDA umbrella for transcatheter closure of patent ductus arteriosus. Circulation 1994;90:2525–2528.

183. Bullock AM, Menahern S, Wilkinson JL. Infective endocarditis on an occluder closing an atrial septal defect. Cardiol Young 1999;9:65–67.

184. Goldstein JA, Beardslee MA, Xu H, et al. Infective endocarditis resulting from CardioSEAL closure of a patent foramen ovale. Catheter Cardiovasc Interv 2002;55:217–220.

185. Foster E, Kusumoto FM, Sobol SM, Schiller NB. Streptococcal endocarditis temporally related to transesophageal echocardiography. J Am Soc Echocardiogr 1990;3:424–427.

186. Moriyama Y, Toyohira H, Saigenji H, et al. Infective mitral valve endocarditis after percutaneous transvenous mitral commissurotomy. Eur J Cardiothorac Surg 1995;9:111–112.

187. Park S, Montoya A, Moreno N, et al. Infective aortic endocarditis after percutaneous balloon aortic valvuloplasty. Ann Thorac Surg 1993;56:1161–1162.

188. Shrivastava S, Agarwal R. Infective endocarditis after balloon mitral dilatation. Int J Cardiol 1992;36:373.

189. Kalra GS, Wander GS, Anand IS. Right sided endocarditis after balloon dilatation of the pulmonary valve. Br Heart J 1990;63:368–369.

190. Cujec B, McMeekin J, Lopez J. Bacterial endocarditis after percutaneous aortic valvuloplasty. Am Heart J 1988;115:178–179.

191. Sanyal SK, Wilson N, Twum-Danso K, et al. *Moraxella* endocarditis following balloon angioplasty of aortic coarctation. Am Heart J 1990;119:1421–1423.

192. Aziz S, Palmer N, Newall N, Ramsdale DR. Bacteraemia following complex percutaneous coronary intervention. TCT Meeting 2003, Washington, USA. Am J Cardiol 2003;64(Suppl):112L.

193. Palmer ND, Ramsdale DR. Mitral valve endocarditis resulting from coagulase-negative *Staphylococcus* after stent implantation in a saphenous vein graft. Cardiol Rev 2005;13:152–154.

194. Grech V, Sammut P, Parascandolo R. Bacterial endocarditis following lacrimal duct probing. J Pediatr Ophthalmol Strabismus 2001;38:49–50.

195. Haas AF, Grekin RC. Antibiotic prophylaxis in dermatologic surgery. J Am Acad Dermatol 1995;32:155–176.

196. Flanagan PG, Carmichael A. Endocarditis following skin procedures. J Infect 1993;27:341–342.

197. Paterson P, Dunn KW. Bacterial endocarditis following minor burn injury. Case report and review. Burns 1999;25:515–517.

198. Apple J, Hunt JL, Wait M, Purdue G. Delayed presentations of aortic valve endocarditis in patients with thermal injury. J Trauma 2002;52:406–409.

199. Nambiar P, Ratnatunga C. Prosthetic valve endocarditis in a patient with Marfan's syndrome following acupuncture. J Heart Valve Dis 2001;10:689–690.

200. Scheel O, Sundsfjord A, Lunde P, Andersen BM. Endocarditis after acupuncture and injection—treatment by a natural healer. JAMA 1992;267:56.

201. Ramage IJ, Wilson N, Thomson RB. Fashion victim: infective endocarditis after nasal piercing. Arch Dis Child 1997;77:187.

202. Tronel H, Chaudemanche H, Pechier N, et al. Endocarditis due to *Neisseria mucosa* after tongue piercing. Clin Microbiol Infect 2001;7:275–276.

203. Ochsenfahrt C, Friedl R, Hannekun A, Schumacher BA. Endocarditis after nipple piercing in a patient with a bicuspid aortic valve. Ann Thorac Surg 2001;71:1365–1366.

204. Satchithananda DK, Walsh J, Schofield PM. Bacterial endocarditis following repeated tattooing. Heart 2001;85:11–12.

205. Horstkotte D, Follath F, Gutschik E, et al. The Task Force on Infective Endocarditis of the European Society of Cardiology. Guidelines on Prevention, Diagnosis and Treatment of Infective Endocarditis. Full Text. Eur Heart J 2004; 1–37. www.escardio.org.

206. Littler WA. Clindamycin suspension and endocarditis prophylaxis. Br Dent J 2001;190:407.

207. Wilson AP. Antibiotic prophylaxis in cardiac surgery. J Antimicrob Chemother 1988;21:522–524.

CHAPTER 6

Treatment: Antimicrobial Therapy

GENERAL MANAGEMENT

An algorithm for the management of patients with infective endocarditis is shown in Figure 6.1.

General principles and specific guidelines for medical treatment have been published in the UK, Europe, and the USA [1–8].

Infective endocarditis requires prompt treatment with appropriate antimicrobial drugs, administered parenterally in doses sufficient to eradicate the organism from the blood, from vegetations and from local or metastatic foci of infection. Parenteral administration ensures complete bioavailability, high serum concentrations, and good penetration into the vegetation. Treatment should begin immediately after blood cultures have been taken—especially in patients with severe sepsis, severe valvular dysfunction, conduction disturbance or embolic events, and should be adjusted once the organism has been identified and the antibiotic sensitivities are known.

The type and duration of antimicrobial treatment is based on the organism responsible, its sensitivity, a history of penicillin allergy, and whether the valve involved is a native or a prosthetic valve [7,8]. Advice from the microbiologist should be sought. Organisms exist at very high densities inside vegetations (10^9–10^{10} per gram) protected from host defenses and cure requires sterilization of vegetations with bactericidal agents in high concentrations for long enough [9,10]. Generally, bactericidal therapy requires a combination of antimicrobials with synergistic activity such as a cell-wall-active agent (B-lactams and glycopeptides) and an aminoglycoside.

Antibiotics That May Be Used in Treatment

Benzylpenicillin remains an important and useful antibiotic but is inactivated by bacterial beta-lactamases.

Penicillinase-resistant penicillins such as flucloxacillin are not inactivated by the enzyme and may be used in the treatment of penicillin-resistant staphylococci.

Broad-spectrum penicillins including ampicillin and amoxicillin are active against certain Gram-positive and Gram-negative organisms but are inactivated by penicillinases produced by *Staphylococcus aureus* and by common Gram-negative bacilli such as *Escherichia coli*. Co-amoxiclav consists of amoxicillin with the beta-lactamase inhibitor clavulanic acid and can be of use in beta-lactamase-producing bacteria that are resistant to amoxicillin.

Antipseudomonal penicillins include the carboxypenicillin ticarcillin and are principally indicated for infection with *Pseudomonas aeruginosa* and certain other Gram-negative bacilli including *Proteus* spp. Ticarcillin is available in combination with clavulanic acid (Timentin), which is active against beta-lactamase-producing bacteria resistant to ticarcillin. The ureidopenicillin piperacillin is more active than ticarcillin against *P. aeruginosa*. Tazocin (piperacillin with the beta-lactamase inhibitor tazobactam) is active against beta-lactamase-producing bacteria resistant to the ureidopenicillins. Its spectrum of activity is comparable to the carbapenems, imipenem and meropenem. These agents should be given with an aminoglycoside since they have synergistic effects.

"Third-generation" cephalosporins such as cefotaxime, ceftazidime, and ceftriaxone have greater activity

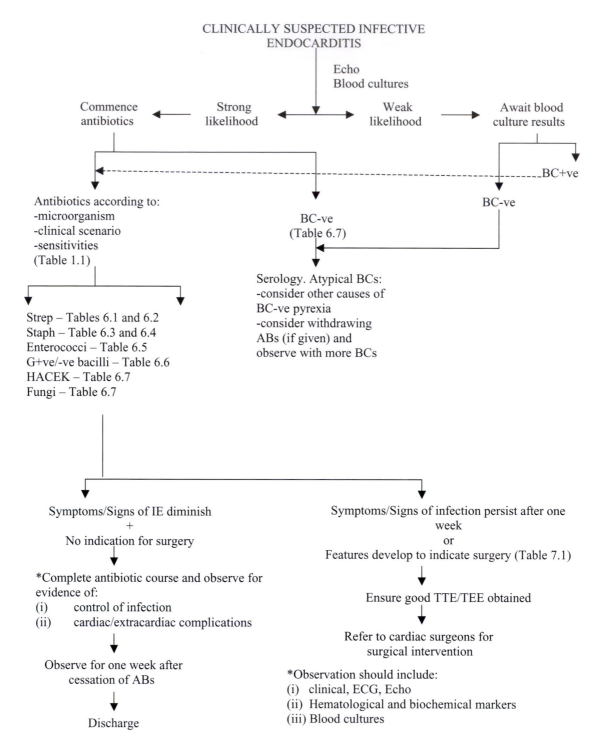

CLINICALLY SUSPECTED INFECTIVE
ENDOCARDITIS

Echo
Blood cultures

Commence   Strong   Weak   Await blood
antibiotics   likelihood   likelihood   culture results

BC+ve

BC-ve

Antibiotics according to:
-microorganism
-clinical scenario
-sensitivities
(Table 1.1)

BC-ve
(Table 6.7)

Strep – Tables 6.1 and 6.2
Staph – Table 6.3 and 6.4
Enterococci – Table 6.5
G+ve/-ve bacilli – Table 6.6
HACEK – Table 6.7
Fungi – Table 6.7

Serology. Atypical BCs:
-consider other causes of
BC-ve pyrexia
-consider withdrawing
ABs (if given) and
observe with more BCs

Symptoms/Signs of IE diminish
+
No indication for surgery

Symptoms/Signs of infection persist after one
week
or
Features develop to indicate surgery (Table 7.1)

*Complete antibiotic course and observe for
evidence of:
(i)   control of infection
(ii)   cardiac/extracardiac complications

Ensure good TTE/TEE obtained

Refer to cardiac surgeons for
surgical intervention

Observe for one week after
cessation of ABs

*Observation should include:
(i) clinical, ECG, Echo
(ii) Hematological and biochemical markers
(iii) Blood cultures

Discharge

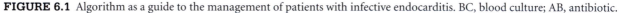

FIGURE 6.1 Algorithm as a guide to the management of patients with infective endocarditis. BC, blood culture; AB, antibiotic.

than the "second-generation" cefuroxime and cefamandole against certain Gram-negative bacteria but are less active against *Staphylococcus aureus*. Ceftazidime has good activity against *P. aeruginosa* and other Gram-negative bacteria and ceftriaxone has a longer half-life and only needs once daily administration. Cefoxitin, a cephamycin antibiotic, is active against *Bacteroides fragilis*.

Beta-lactam antibiotics include aztreonam, imipenem, and meropenem. Aztreonam is a monocyclic beta-lactam (monobactam) antibiotic active against Gram-negative aerobic bacteria including *P. aeruginosa*, *Neisseria meningitidis*, and *Haemophilus influenzae*. It is inactive against Gram-positive organisms. Imipenem, a carbapenem, has a broad spectrum of activity against many aerobic and anaerobic Gram-positive and Gram-negative bacteria. Since it is partially inactivated in the kidney by enzymatic activity, it is administered in combination with cilastin, a specific enzyme inhibitor that blocks its renal metabolism. Meropenem is similar to imipenem but is stable to the renal enzyme that inactivates imipenem and therefore can be used without cilastin.

Aminoglycosides include amikacin, gentamicin, streptomycin, and tobramycin. All are bactericidal and active against some Gram-positive and many Gram-negative organisms. Amikacin, gentamicin, and tobramycin are also active against *P. aeruginosa*. Serum concentration monitoring avoids both excessive and subtherapeutic concentrations, thus preventing toxicity and ensuring efficacy. In patients with normal renal function, aminoglycoside concentrations should be measured after three or four doses, but they should be measured earlier and more frequently in those with renal impairment. Blood samples should be taken 1 hour after IV administration (peak) and just before the next dose (trough). Gentamicin has a broad spectrum but is inactive against anaerobes and has poor activity against hemolytic streptococci and pneumococci. It should be used in combination with another antibiotic such as penicillin. The dose is up to 5 mg/kg daily in divided doses every 8 hours. Loading doses and maintenance may be calculated on the basis of the patient's weight, using a nomogram. Adjustments are then made according to serum gentamicin concentrations. In staphylococcal endocarditis, gentamicin is given in conventional doses to achieve a "peak" concentration of 5–10 mg/L and a "trough" level of <2 mg/L. Amikacin is more stable than gentamicin to enzyme inactivation and may be used for serious infections caused by gentamicin-resistant Gram-negative bacilli. Tobramycin is similar to gentamicin but is slightly more active against *P. aeruginosa*.

Macrolide antibiotics include erythromycin and clarithromycin. Erythromycin has an antibacterial spectrum that is similar to penicillin and is an alternative in penicillin-allergic patients. Azithromycin is a macrolide with slightly less activity against Gram-positive bacteria but enhanced activity against some Gram-negative bacteria such as *H. influenzae*. It has a long tissue half-life and once daily dosage is recommended. Clarithromycin is an erythromycin derivative with greater activity than erythromycin. Tissue concentrations are higher than with erythromycin and it is given twice daily.

Clindamycin is active against Gram-positive cocci, including penicillin-resistant staphylococci, and also against many anaerobic bacteria, especially *Bacteroides fragilis*.

Fusidic acid may be used for staphylococci, especially penicillin-resistant staphylococci, although a second antistaphylococcal antibiotic is required to prevent emergence of resistance.

The glycopeptide antibiotics vancomycin and teicoplanin have bactericidal activity against aerobic and anaerobic Gram-positive bacteria. Vancomycin is used for treating Gram-positive cocci including multiresistant staphylococci. There are increasing reports of vancomycin-resistant enterococci (VRE). It has a long duration of action and can be given 12-hourly. Teicoplanin is similar but has a longer duration of action and can be given once daily.

Linezolid, an oxazolidinone antibacterial, is active against Gram-positive bacteria including methicillin-resistant *Staphylococcus aureus* (MRSA) and VRE. It should be reserved for treating organisms resistant to other antibacterials or when they are poorly tolerated. It is inactive against Gram-negative organisms.

Synercid—a combination of the streptogramin antibiotics quinupristin and dalfopristin—may be useful for Gram-positive bacterial endocarditis with MRSA or for patients who cannot be treated with other agents. It is not active against *Enterococcus faecalis*.

Pharmacokinetic Issues

For antimicrobials with time-dependent bactericidal activity (B-lactams and glycopeptides), it is necessary to attain concentrations persistently above the MIC (see below), in both serum and vegetations. This justifies the use of high doses, despite their time-dependent activity, especially for teicoplanin in staphylococcal endocarditis, or ceftriaxone in endocarditis due to Gram-negative aerobic bacilli.

For antimicrobials with concentration-dependent bactericidal activity, high peak concentrations must be obtained. A post-antibiotic effect (PAE) observed in Gram-negative endocarditis allows an increased interval between doses, but this does not apply for Gram-positive, mainly enterococcal endocarditis, for which no PAE has been shown in vivo.

Dosing Regimens

For B-lactams and glycopeptides with time-dependent activity and no PAE, serum levels must be maintained throughout the dosing interval to prevent regrowth of bacteria between doses. This interval is determined by the rate of drug elimination and the serum half-life. Benzylpenicillin and anti-staphylococcal penicillins should be administered every 3–4 hours. Ceftriaxone, which has a long serum half-life (8 hours), can be administered once a day in the case of highly susceptible organisms such as viridans streptococci. Vancomycin and teicoplanin are administered every 12 or 24 hours respectively after a loading dose for teicoplanin because of its long half-life. Aminoglycosides can be administered twice a day for Gram-negative bacilli endocarditis, but are needed three times daily for Gram-positive and enterococcal endocarditis.

Maximizing Effectiveness of Antimicrobial Treatment

In evaluating the potential efficacy of an antibiotic, the minimal inhibitory concentration (MIC) must be considered [11]. The MIC is the minimum concentration that inhibits bacterial growth in vitro. With most streptococci or staphylococci, the MIC and minimal bactericidal concentration (MBC) of cell-wall active antibiotics (penicillins, cephalosporins, and vancomycin) do not differ significantly [12]. However, the MBCs of these antibiotics are much higher than the MICs for a minority of strains of streptococci and staphylococci and for many strains of enterococci. When the difference is 10-fold or more, or when the MBC/MIC ratio is >32, the strains are said to be *tolerant*, which indicates a slower rate of kill [13]. Tolerance can be overcome by addition of an aminoglycoside – resulting in a more rapid bactericidal activity [14–16]. In treatment of enterococcal endocarditis an aminoglycoside must be added to amoxicillin or ampicillin to obtain adequate bactericidal effect and cure, although this is probably not essential in tolerant streptococcal or staphylococcal infection [17–20]. Serum drug level monitoring during aminoglycoside therapy is recommended. Gentamicin peak serum concentration (1 hour post IV dose) should be 5–10 mg/L but the trough level should be <2.0 mg/L to avoid renal or ototoxic effects. Optimum vancomycin effects are achieved if serum concentrations are kept at least 2–4 times above the MIC of the causative organism. Trough levels should be 10–15 mg/L.

The necessary frequency of dosing varies, depending on the organism and the antimicrobial(s) being used and whether or not a post-antibiotic effect exists. Intravenous antibiotics should be commenced as soon as the diagnosis is made and after appropriate blood culture samples have been collected and sent to the microbiology laboratory. Initially, IV benzylpenicillin and gentamicin in the

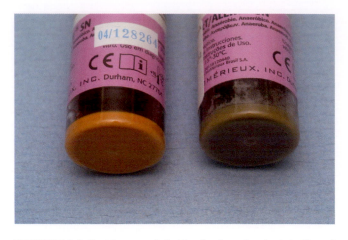

FIGURE 6.2 Positive growth in blood culture bottles is indicated by a color change from green (right) to yellow (left).

same dosage as for treatment of IE caused by penicillin-sensitive viridans streptococci should be used. If there is a strong possibility of staphylococcal infection, e.g. IV drug abuse, infected hemodialysis lines, or pacemaker infection, IV flucloxacillin and/or vancomycin should be used instead of benzylpenicillin. Once the blood culture results are known, the treatment can be modified and a decision made about its duration (Figure 6.2). An exception to this might be in patients recently receiving antibiotics, when delaying treatment for a few days can increase the chance of isolating the responsible organism on subsequent blood cultures. Such delay is only reasonable in closely monitored patients with subacute illness who have no evidence of severe or progressive valve dysfunction, heart failure, or embolic complications.

Isolation of the infecting organism is extremely important, so that an appropriate antimicrobial agent can be chosen and the antimicrobial susceptibility of the organism established. Both MIC and MBC may be useful, although no data suggest that MBC is any better than the more simple and reproducible MIC test. Therefore, routine determination of MBC or serum bactericidal level is not recommended [21].

A peak serum bactericidal titer (the highest dilution of the patient's serum whilst receiving antibiotics that kills a standard inoculum of the patient's organism in vitro and measured by back-titration) of 1:8 or greater usually indicates an adequate therapeutic effect. A peak bactericidal titer of 1:64 and a trough of 1:32 has been reported to represent optimal therapy [22]. Determination of the titer is valuable only when response to treatment with the recommended regimens is suboptimal, when IE is due to an unusual organism, or when an unconventional treatment regimen is used [18]. However, caution should be used when using titer data, in order to avoid false reassurance

TABLE 6.1 Treatment of infective endocarditis due to penicillin-sensitive viridans streptococci and *S. bovis* (MIC <0.1 mg/L) in adults

Antibiotic	Dose/route	Duration
Benzylpenicillin	7.2–12 g IV daily in 4–6 divided doses	4–6 weeks[b]
+ gentamicin[a]	3–5 mg/kg IV daily in 2–3 divided doses (max 240 mg)	2 weeks[c]
Benzylpenicillin	7.2–12 g IV daily in 4–6 divided doses	2 weeks[d]
+ gentamicin[a]	3–5 mg/kg IV daily in 2–3 divided doses (max 240 mg)	2 weeks
Teicoplanin [172]	400 mg IV bolus 12-hourly for first 3 doses, then 400 mg IV daily[e]	4 weeks
Ceftriaxone	2 g/day IV	4 weeks
For those patients allergic to penicillin		
Vancomycin	30 mg/kg IV in 24 h in 2 divided doses[f] (infused over 2 h)	4 weeks
+ gentamicin[a]	3–5 mg/kg IV daily in 2–3 divided doses (max 240 mg)	2 weeks

[a] Loading dose and maintenance dose of gentamicin may be calculated on the basis of the patient's age, weight and renal function using a nomogram, with appropriate adjustments in dose being made according to serum gentamicin concentrations.
 With renal impairment, dose may be reduced according to creatinine clearance using Mawer nomogram or to blood urea levels, e.g.
  7–17 mmol/L: 80 mg 12-hourly
  17–33 mmol/L: 80 mg daily
  >33 mmol/L: 80 mg alternate days.
Serum gentamicin levels should be checked twice per week if serum creatinine is normal and more often if elevated.
Ideally:
  Pre(trough) level (taken just prior to dose) <2 mg/L
  If >2 mg/L – drug interval must be increased or dose reduced
  Peak level (taken 1 hour after IV dose) < 10 mg/L Preferably 3–5 mg/L
  If level exceeds this – reduce dose.
[b] Duration adjusted according to clinical response and advice from microbiologist.
[c] Four weeks of benzylpenicillin alone for sensitive streptococci may be a useful option for the elderly or those with existing hearing impairment or poor renal function.
[d] Conditions to be met for a 2 week treatment regimen for viridans streptococci and *S. bovis* endocarditis:
  Penicillin-sensitive viridans streptococci including *S. bovis* (penicillin MIC <0.1 mg/L)
  No cardiovascular risk factors, e.g. heart failure, aortic or mitral regurgitation, conduction abnormalities
  No evidence of thromboembolism
  Native valve infection
  No vegetations >5 mm diameter demonstrated on echocardiography
  Clinical response within 7 days including abolition of pyrexia.
[e] Serum teicoplanin levels should be checked to ensure appropriate blood concentrations.
[f] Serum trough level of vancomycin should be maintained between 10 and 15 mg/L to ensure optimal efficacy.

of microbiological efficacy despite the lack of evidence of clinical improvement.

TREATMENT REGIMENS FOR SPECIFIC MICROORGANISMS

Streptococci and Staphylococci
The majority (80%) of NVE is caused by viridans streptococci (50–70%), *Staphylococcus aureus* (25%), and enterococci (10%) [23–30]. Certain organisms are more frequently associated with particular clinical situations and procedures (see Table 1.1). For example, *S. aureus* is the most frequent cause of endocarditis in IV drug abusers (60%), in insulin-dependent diabetes mellitus, and in infection of the tricuspid valve, and this microorganism is particularly destructive [27,29]. *S. epidermidis* more often causes indolent infection on previously damaged valves [25,31].

Regimens for treatment of streptococci are shown in Tables 6.1 and 6.2 and for staphylococci in Tables 6.3 and 6.4 [5,6,8,18,25,32–34].

Treatment of streptococcal endocarditis depends on the clinical complexity of the infection in the individual patient and on the antibiotic susceptibility of the organism (Figures 6.3 and 6.4). For example, in uncomplicated IE caused by fully penicillin-sensitive viridans streptococci or *S. bovis* (MIC <0.1 mg/L) on a native valve, treatment for 2 weeks with IV benzylpenicillin + gentamicin is generally sufficient to cure the infection. Whereas, if there is any evidence of cardiac or embolic complications or if the organism is less sensitive to penicillin (MIC between 0.1 mg/L and 0.5 mg/L), benzylpenicillin should be continued for 4–6 weeks with gentamicin for the first 2 weeks. For more resistant streptococci (MIC >0.5 mg/L), treatment with gentamicin for longer may be necessary, although the risk of ototoxicity increases.

Frequent dosing of penicillin is necessary as the initial high peak concentration rapidly decreases due to glomerular filtration, tubular excretion in the kidney, and inactivation of penicillin (half-life 20–30 minutes) in blood. Although prolonged courses of antibiotics probably produce more effective outcomes, on the whole,

TABLE 6.2 Treatment of infective endocarditis due to penicillin-relative resistant viridans streptococci and *S. bovis* (MIC > 0.1 mg/L) in adults

Antibiotic	Dose/route	Duration
Benzylpenicillin	12–14 g IV daily in 4–6 divided doses	4–6 weeks[b]
+ gentamicin[a]	3–5 mg/kg IV daily in 2–3 divided doses (max 240 mg)	2 weeks[b]
or		
Teicoplanin[c]	400 mg IV bolus 12-hourly for 3 doses, then 400 mg IV daily	4 weeks[b]
+ gentamicin[a]	3–5 mg/kg IV daily in 2–3 divided doses (max 240 mg)	2 weeks[b]
For those patients allergic to penicillin		
Vancomycin[d]	30 mg/kg IV per 24 h in 2 divided doses (infused over 2 hrs)	4 weeks[b]
+ gentamicin[a]	3–5 mg/kg IV daily in 2–3 divided doses (max 240 mg)	2 weeks[b]

[a] See Table 6.1.
[b] Duration adjusted according to clinical response and advice from microbiologist.
[c] Serum teicoplanin levels should be checked to ensure appropriate blood concentrations.
[d] As a guide the dose may be adjusted to achieve 1 hour post-infusion serum concentrations of about 30 mg/L and trough concentrations of 10–15 mg/L, although the correlation between peak and trough levels with toxicity and efficacy is not high.

S. pneumoniae—treat as penicillin-sensitive viridans streptococci but check sensitivity as penicillin-resistant pneumococci are now being isolated.
S. pyogenes—(group A streptococci), groups B, C, and G streptococci—treat as per penicillin-sensitive viridans streptococci [173].
S. adjacens and *S. defectivus* (nutritionally variant streptococci)—treat with either benzylpenicillin/gentamicin combination or vancomycin and gentamicin regimen. Advice from microbiologist should be sought.

TABLE 6.3 Treatment of endocarditis due to staphylococci on native valve

Antibiotic	Dose/route	Duration
Penicillin-sensitive (non-B-lactamase producers)		
Benzylpenicillin	12–14 g IV daily in 4–6 divided doses	6 weeks
+ gentamicin[a]	3–5 mg/kg IV daily in 2–3 divided doses	3–5 days
Methicillin-sensitive staphylococci (B-lactamase producer)		
Flucloxacillin	8–12 g IV daily in 4 divided doses	6 weeks
+ gentamicin[a]	3–5 mg/kg IV daily in 2–3 divided doses	3–5 days
For those patients allergic to penicillin		
Vancomycin	30 mg/kg IV in 24 hours in 2 divided doses (infused over 2 h)	6 weeks
+ gentamicin[a]	3–5 mg/kg IV daily in 2–3 divided doses	3–5 days
Methicillin-resistant staphylococci[b]		
Vancomycin	30 mg/kg IV in 24 hours in 2 divided doses (infused over 2 h)	6 weeks
+ gentamicin[a] [174]	3–5 mg/kg IV daily in 2–3 divided doses	3–5 days

[a] Gentamicin blood levels must be checked 2–3 times in this week period.
See Table 6.1. Peak levels 5–10 mg/L.
Oral Fusidic acid may be considered as an alternative to gentamicin for combination treatment for fusidic acid-sensitive strains [175–177].
Rifampicin may be added to the penicillin, gentamicin, or vancomycin regimens for poor responders.
In some patients with uncomplicated tricuspid valve endocarditis due to IV drug abuse, 2 weeks of IV flucloxacillin and gentamicin for methicillin-sensitive staphylococcal infection is often effective (see text).
[b] Linezolid or Synercid may be used in MRSA.

TABLE 6.4 Treatment of endocarditis due to staphylococci on prosthetic valve or other prosthetic material

Antibiotic	Dose/route	Duration
Methicillin-sensitive staphylococci		
Flucloxacillin	8–12 g IV daily in 4 divided doses	6 weeks
+ rifampicin[a]	300 mg orally 8-hourly	6 weeks
+ gentamicin[b]	3–5 mg/kg IV daily in 2–3 divided doses	2 weeks
Methicillin-resistant staphylococci[c]		
Vancomycin	30 mg/kg IV in 24 h in 2 divided doses (infused over 2 h)	6 weeks
+ rifampicin[a]	300 mg orally 8-hourly	6 weeks
+ gentamicin[b]	3–5 mg/kg IV daily in 2–3 divided doses	2 weeks

[a] Resistance to rifampicin develops rapidly and therefore should never be given alone. Fluoroquinolones are an alternative to rifampicin if the microorganism is resistant to rifampicin.
[b] See Table 6.1. Peak levels 5–10 mg/L.
[c] This regimen may be used if patient is allergic to penicillin.

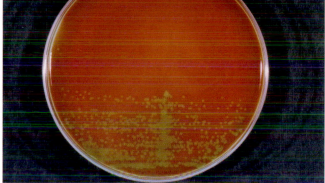

FIGURE 6.3 Colonies of viridans streptococci appear to have a greenish tinge when grown on a blood agar plate.

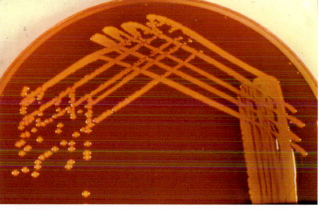

FIGURE 6.5 Blood agar plate showing the large, gold-colored colonies of *Staphylococcus aureus* grown in blood culture bottles from a patient with infective endocarditis of the aortic valve. Courtesy of Dr Lisa Grech.

there is limited evidence that 4 weeks is better than 3, or that 6 weeks is better than 5 weeks. As indicated above, some cases of endocarditis can be cured by only 2 weeks' treatment, for example in uncomplicated, penicillin-sensitive, streptococcal native valve endocarditis (see Table 6.1) and drug addicts with *S. aureus* tricuspid valve endocarditis. It is thought that combining penicillin/flucloxacillin with gentamicin results in a more rapid defervescence and clearance of bacteremia and this is therefore recommended, although superiority over penicillin alone has not been demonstrated in a clinical trial. Teicoplanin is an alternative to penicillin in streptococcal endocarditis, when the

starting dose should be at least 10 mg/kg and the serum levels checked in order to ensure appropriate blood concentrations. Vancomycin is also an effective alternative to penicillin and the drug of choice in patients allergic to penicillin [2,35]. Ceftriaxone has an excellent pharmacokinetic profile for treating streptococcal IE and may be useful in patients over 65 years or with renal or auditory nerve impairment [36–42].

Staphylococcal IE is a particularly severe and life-threatening infection responsible for about one third of all cases (Figures 6.5–6.8). Early treatment is the key to improving overall prognosis. Ninety percent are due to coagulase-positive *S. aureus* and 10% to coagulase-negative staphylococci. The tube coagulase test or the coagulase spot test is used to distinguish between the two

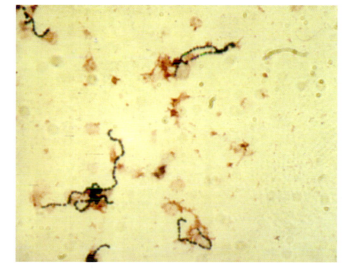

FIGURE 6.4 Gram-positive streptococci seen microscopically are arranged in a "chain" formation. Courtesy of Dr Lisa Grech.

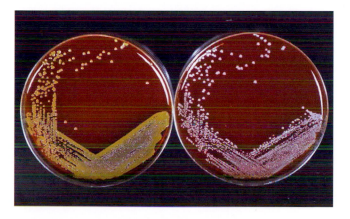

FIGURE 6.6 Two blood agar plates showing the contrast between the golden yellow colonies of *Staphylococcus aureus* (left) and the white colonies of *Staphylococcus epidermidis* (right).

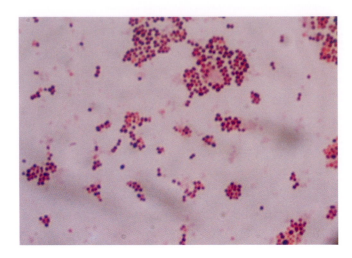

FIGURE 6.7 Gram-positive staphylococci – microscopic appearance.

major species of pathogenic staphylococci (Figures 6.9 and 6.10).

S. aureus is the only common cause of acute endocarditis and can attack normal hearts in staphylococcal septicemia. The organism predominantly affects left-sided valves except in IV drug abusers. Less than 10% of S. aureus strains are susceptible to penicillin although community-acquired strains are frequently methicillin-sensitive. Methicillin-resistant S. aureus (MRSA) accounts for approximately 50% of cases of S. aureus endocarditis in drug abusers and endocarditis acquired in hospitals,

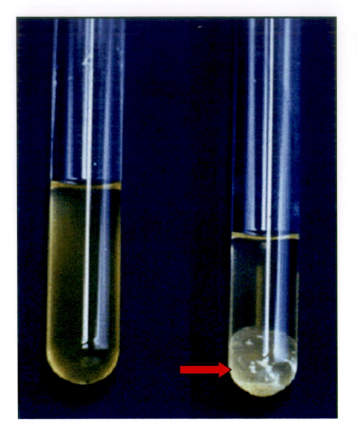

FIGURE 6.9 The tube coagulase test tests the ability of the staphylococcal strain to produce a thrombin-like enzyme, coagulase. After incubating diluted plasma and a broth culture of the organism, formation of a clot (arrow) within the tube (right), but not in a control tube (left), indicates that the organism is coagulase positive.

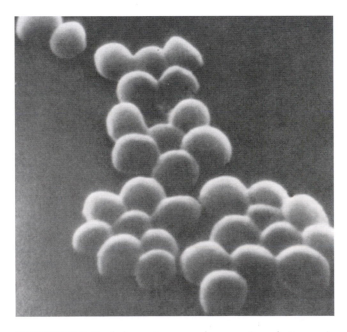

FIGURE 6.8 Staphylococci as seen by scanning electron microscopy.

e.g. IV access site infection or transvenous pacemaker infection [43,44]. Methicillin-resistant S. epidermidis is responsible for most cases of S. epidermidis endocarditis on prosthetic valves but uncommonly causes native valve endocarditis [44–46]. When it does, it usually presents a subacute picture. Treatment of suspected methicillin-resistant staphylococcal endocarditis in these situations or of proven infection must include vancomycin. Rifampicin has been used as a supplement to therapy with a penicillin, cephalosporin or vancomycin with or without aminoglycosides in patients responding poorly to these agents [47,48]. Rifampicin is actively taken up by granulocytes and becomes effective against intracellular staphylococci and staphylococci within abscesses. Other agents such as linezolid and Synercid may be alternative choices for infection with MRSA. The emergence of vancomycin intermediate resistance S. aureus (VISA) among MRSA isolates is of great concern; many of these organisms are also resistant to teicoplanin and are called glycopeptide intermediate resistance S. aureus (GISA) [49].

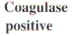

**Coagulase
negative**

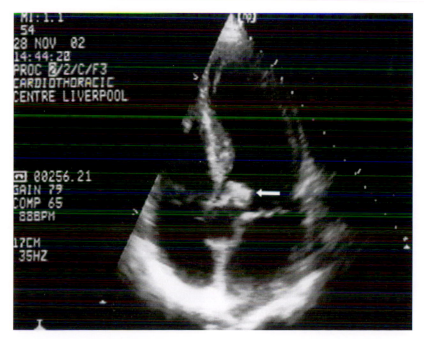

**Coagulase
positive**

FIGURE 6.10 The slide "coagulase" test has the advantage of being faster and simpler to use. Here, coagulase-positive staphylococci produce coagulase which when mixed with plasma on a slide, triggers clotting and causes the plasma to form clump-like clots. The lower slide shows clotted plasma, the upper slide being smooth and unclotted.

Although coagulase-negative staphylococci are the most common cause of PVE, they also affect patients with mitral valve prolapse. Here the course is typically indolent with a good response to medical or surgical treatment. However, *Staphylococcus lugdunensis* is particularly virulent and causes high rates of perivalvular extension of

infection and metastatic seeding to distant organs [49–52]. Such patients require careful observation for the development of such complications.

The *routine* use of back-titrations of the patient's serum against the organism is not recommended for monitoring antibiotic treatment.

Nutritionally Variant Streptococci
These bacteria account for 5–6% of streptococcal endocarditis and are an important cause of culture-negative endocarditis [53]. *Streptococcus adjacens* and *Streptococcus defectivus* appear to be the predominant species. These organisms are residents of the oral cavity, genitourinary and intestinal mucosae. Endocarditis occurs in the setting of prior valvular disease and is characterized by a slow indolent course [53,54]. Morbidity and mortality exceed those of other forms of viridans streptococci and even enterococci [54]. Bacteriological diagnosis may require special techniques [55].

More than 30% of strains are relatively resistant to penicillin and either a penicillin/aminoglycoside combination or vancomycin regimen is usually necessary [55].

Enterococci
E. faecalis accounts for 10% of cases of endocarditis and 90% of all enterococcal endocarditis [56]. Other species that may be responsible include *E. faecium* and *E. durans*. *E. faecalis* endocarditis is most often found in elderly patients and is usually associated with malignancy or manipulation of the gastrointestinal or genitourinary tract (Figures 6.11–6.13). It often produces a subacute rather

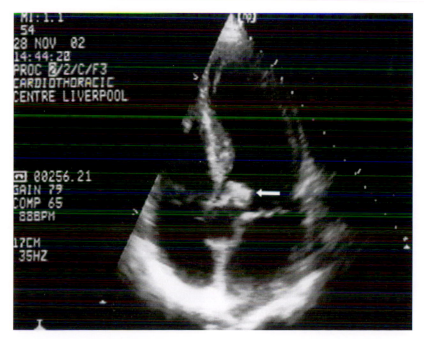

FIGURE 6.11 Echocardiogram showing aortic valve endocarditis and a large vegetation (arrow). The infective endocarditis was due to *Enterococcus faecalis* in a patient with carcinoma of the colon (see Figure 6.12).

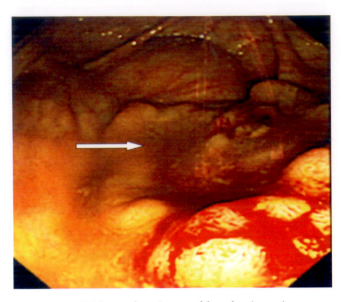

FIGURE 6.12 Ulcerated carcinoma of the colon (arrow) as seen at colonoscopy in a patient who developed *Enterococcus faecalis* aortic valve endocarditis.

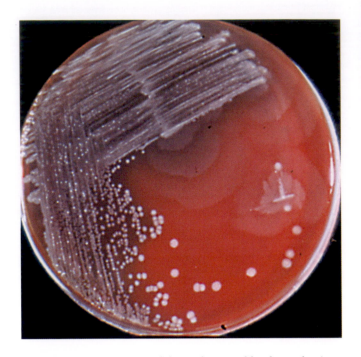

FIGURE 6.14 *Proteus mirabilis* seen here on a blood agar plate is an unusual cause of infective endocarditis seen in patients with severe urinary sepsis and in immunocompromised patients undergoing long-term ventilation on intensive care units.

than an acute endocarditis. These microorganisms are usually more resistant to penicillin than viridans streptococci and relatively resistant to aminoglycosides [57–60]. Some enterococci are multiresistant to antibiotics including vancomycin (VRE) [61,62]. Regimens for treatment are shown in Table 6.5 [18–20,63–64].

First-line treatment is with a synergistic bactericidal combination of IV amoxicillin + gentamicin. Gentamicin-resistant (MIC >500 mg/L) enterococci may not respond to this combination but some strains may respond to high-dose amoxicillin for 6 weeks or to a combination of amoxicillin + streptomycin. Amoxicillin-resistant strains can be treated with a combination of vancomycin (or teicoplanin) and gentamicin and this regimen may be suitable for

patients who are allergic to penicillin. For VRE, linezolid may be useful, while Synercid may be used in vancomycin-resistant *E. faecium*.

Gram-positive and Gram-negative Bacilli

Gram-positive (e.g. *Listeria monocytogenes* and *Proprionibacterium acnes*) and Gram-negative bacilli (e.g. *E. coli*, *Klebsiella* spp., *Serratia* spp., *P. aeruginosa*, *Proteus mirabilis*) are uncommon but serious causes of endocarditis [65–73] (Figure 6.14). Regimens for treatment are shown in Table 6.6 [74–87]. As susceptibility of these organisms is often unpredictable, treatment should be based on susceptibility testing.

Anaerobic Gram-negative bacilli (e.g. *Fusobacterium* spp., *Bacteroides* spp.) require specific treatment which includes high-dose IV penicillin, imipenem, and the addition of metronidazole 500 mg 8-hourly for 6–8 weeks [87,88].

HACEK Group

In recent years, the HACEK group of organisms (*Haemophilus*, *Actinobacillus*, *Cardiobacterium*, *Eikenella*, and *Kingella* species) have become important causes of endocarditis (Figures 6.15 and 6.16), causing large vegetations (>1 cm), large vessel emboli, and congestive cardiac failure [89–98]. This group of organisms will often require 7–21 days of incubation in 10% CO_2 to allow growth. The treatment is shown in Table 6.7 [98–103].

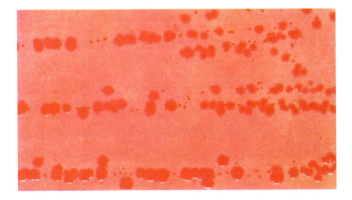

FIGURE 6.13 MacConkey medium. *Enterococcus faecalis* grows as small pinpoint bright magenta-colored colonies. *Escherichia coli* form larger pink colonies.

TABLE 6.5 Treatment of infective endocarditis due to enterococci in adults

Antibiotic	Dose/route	Duration
Gentamicin-sensitive or low-level resistant organism (MIC <500 mg/L)		
Benzylpenicillin	10–12 g IV daily in 4–6 divided doses	4–6 weeks[a]
or ampicillin or amoxicillin	12 g IV daily in 4 divided doses	4–6 weeks[a]
+ gentamicin[b]	3–5 mg/kg IV daily in 2–3 divided doses	4–6 weeks[a]
For those patients allergic to penicillin		
Vancomycin[c]	30 mg/kg IV per 24 h in 2 divided doses (infused over 2 h)	4–6 weeks[a]
+ gentamicin[b]	3–5 mg/kg IV daily in 2–3 divided doses	4–6 weeks[a]

[a] Six weeks' therapy recommended for patients with symptoms >3 months.
[b] Monitor drug serum levels and renal function. See Table 6.1.
[c] Teicoplanin 10 mg/kg IV bolus 12-hourly for first 6 doses then 10 mg/kg IV daily may be an alternative to vancomycin. Levels should be measured.

For gentamicin-highly resistant strains (MIC >500 mg/L), ampicillin or amoxicillin 12 g IV per day in 6 divided doses or as a continuous infusion for 6 weeks is advisable. If the organism is sensitive to streptomycin this could also be added but dose monitoring is necessary to avoid ototoxicity.
For ampicillin-resistant strains, the vancomycin + gentamicin regimen may be effective.
Vancomycin-resistant enterococci (VRE) may respond to IV linezolid 600 mg infused over 30–120 min every 12 h.
Vancomycin-resistant *E. faecium* may respond to Synercid.
For multiresistant strains, expert advice should be sought from the microbiologist.

FIGURE 6.15 Culture of *Haemophilus* on blood agar shows tiny pinpoint colonies, although the quality of the medium can have an effect on the appearance of the colonies. Courtesy of Dr Lisa Grech.

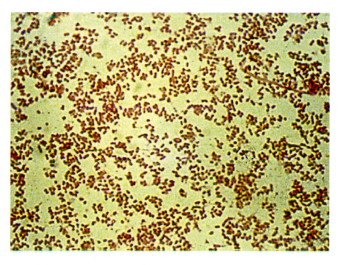

FIGURE 6.16 *Haemophilus* appears microscopically as small, Gram-negative bacilli. Courtesy of Dr Lisa Grech.

Fungi

Fungi, especially *Aspergillus* spp. and *Candida* spp., are also important causes of endocarditis (2–10%), particularly in patients with prosthetic valves, suppressed immunity, or IV drug abuse [104–107]. Patients receiving prolonged, intense antibiotic therapy and hyperalimentation, those with long-term IV catheters in situ, and those with bacterial endocarditis are also at increased risk of fungal endocarditis. Details of the organisms responsible and their sources have been presented by Rubinstein and Lang [108] and are associated with large vegetations and systemic emboli.

Fungal endocarditis demands intensive treatment with potentially toxic agents (Table 6.7). Seventy-five percent of cases are due to *Candida* species and they should be formally identified and sensitivity tested. Patients require careful observation with frequent monitoring of their hematology and biochemistry. Surgery should be performed early after commencing treatment, especially in patients with large vegetations, evidence of emboli, poor response to treatment, *Aspergillus* endocarditis, and in those with prosthetic valves, since mortality is unacceptably high with treatment with antimycotic agents alone [108–110] (Figures 6.17–6.19). However, fungal valvular infection is aggressive and difficult to treat surgically. There is a high risk of embolization and serious perioperative bleeding may occur when infected tissue is resected [111]. Usually surgery is complicated by the need for radical debridement and aortic root reconstruction. Prosthetic valve fungal endocarditis is particularly serious – the first episode is usually a result of nosocomial candidemia, and recurrent episodes are frequent [110,112,113]. In this situation, urgent surgical intervention is recommended and antifungal drug treatment should be continued for life.

TABLE 6.6 Treatment of endocarditis due to Gram-positive and Gram-negative bacilli

Organism	Antibiotic	Dose/route	Duration
Listeria monocytogenes[a]	Amoxicillin	12 g IV daily in 4 divided doses	6 weeks
	+ gentamicin[b]	3–5 mg/kg IV daily in 2–3 divided doses	4–6 weeks
Pseudomonas aeruginosa[a]	Tazocin[c]	18 g IV daily in 6 divided doses	6 weeks
	or ceftazidime	6 g IV daily in 3 divided doses	6 weeks
	or imipenem	2–4 g IV daily in 4 divided doses	6 weeks
	or aztreonam	8 g IV daily in 4 divided doses	6 weeks
	+ gentamicin[b]	3–5 mg/kg IV daily in 2–3 divided doses	4–6 weeks
	or tobramycin	8 mg/kg IV daily in 4 divided doses	4–6 weeks
Enterobacteraceae[d]	Amoxicillin	12 g IV daily in 4 divided doses	6 weeks
	or cefotaxime	8 g IV daily in 4 divided doses	6 weeks
	or imipenem	2–4 g IV daily in 4 divided doses	6 weeks
	or aztreonam	8 g IV daily in 4 divided doses	6 weeks
	+ gentamicin[b]	3–5 mg/kg IV daily in 2–3 divided doses	4–6 weeks

[a] Treatment is usually specific and based on results of antibacterial sensitivity testing [178].
[b] See Table 6.1. Peak levels 5–10 mg/L.
[c] Tazocin (piperacillin + beta-lactamase inhibitor, tazobactam) is probably better than piperacillin alone.
[d] *E. coli/Klebsiella/Enterobacter/Serratia/Proteus*—drug regimen often depends on individual organism, sensitivity testing, and advice from microbiologist.

Amphotericin B has been the single most effective agent but it requires prolonged infusion periods and has unpleasant side effects and adverse effects. Liposomal amphotericin B may be particularly effective in *Aspergillus* endocarditis. Flucytosine is less well defined although most authors recommend a combination of the two agents. FC is toxic to liver and bone marrow and frequent monitoring of blood and liver function tests are mandatory.

Voriconazole is a new antifungal agent which may be useful for serious *Aspergillus* infections.

TABLE 6.7 Treatment of HACEK group, fungal, and culture-negative endocarditis
HACEK group

Antibiotic	Dose/route	Duration
Ampicillin or amoxicillin[a]	12 g IV daily in 4 divided doses	4–6 weeks[b]
+ gentamicin[c]	3–5 mg/kg IV daily in 2–3 divided doses	2 weeks

[a] If amoxicillin-resistant, a third generation cephalosporin such as IV ceftriaxone 2 g/day in a single dose is given for 3–4 weeks in native valve endocarditis and 6 weeks in prosthetic valve endocarditis. It has a long half-life.
[b] 6 weeks for patients with prosthetic valve endocarditis.
[c] See Table 6.1. Peak levels 5–10 mg/L.
Ofloxacin may be useful in *Actinobacillus* endocarditis [179].

Fungi[a]

Antifungal	Dose/route	Duration
Amphotericin B[b]	1 mg/kg IV every 24 h (total dose 2–2.5 g)	6 weeks
± flucytosine[c]	150–200 mg/kg oral per day in 4 divided doses	6 weeks

[a] Current antifungal agents will not cure fungal endocarditis except in rare cases and combined medical treatment and surgical treatment should be employed.
[b] Amphotericin B as a lipid complex or encapsulated in liposomes have been shown to have reduced toxicity enabling much higher doses to be given without substantial side effects [180]. Advice from microbiologist should be sought.
[c] Marrow depression and hepatic necrosis are side effects; plasma concentrations for optimal response are 25–50 mg/L and should not be allowed to exceed 80 mg/L.

Culture-negative[a]

Antibiotic	Dose/route	Duration
Vancomycin	15 mg/kg IV every 12 h	6 weeks
+ gentamicin[b]	3–5mg/kg IV daily in 2–3 divided doses	2 weeks

[a] When serology for atypical organisms such as *Chlamydia*, *Coxiella*, and *Bartonella* are negative.
[b] See Table 6.1. Peak levels 5–10 mg/L.

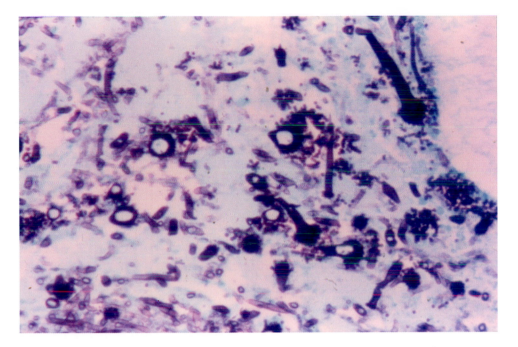

FIGURE 6.17 *Aspergillus* species may be isolated from blood cultures or directly from vegetations or emboli removed surgically. They are recognized by their conidiophores – swollen ends of hyphae from which radiate large numbers of sterigmata (short lengths of narrower hyphae) ending in short chains of spores. Courtesy of Dr Hani Zakhour.

Blood Culture-negative Endocarditis

Treatment should include antibiotics that are appropriate for the most likely organism but should generally cover Gram-positive and Gram-negative organisms (Table 6.7). Early surgical intervention is often necessary [114,115]. Patients with *Coxiella* and *Chlamydia* infection need valve replacement and prolonged treatment since reinfection commonly occurs.

For Q-fever endocarditis, treatment with doxycycline (1 g/day) is indicated for at least 3 years (possibly for life) plus either cotrimoxazole (1.92 g/day), rifampicin (300 mg/day), or ciprofloxacin (1.5 g/day) since the liver is usually chronically infected. Other agents, e.g. ofloxacin, hydroxychloroquine, are being evaluated in combination therapy for Q-fever infection [116]. During treatment, serological testing should be performed monthly for

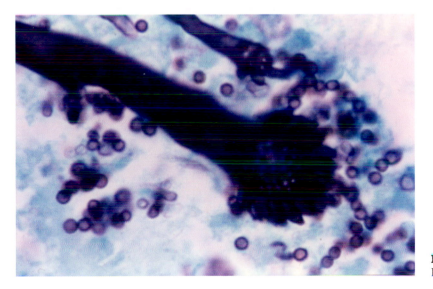

FIGURE 6.18 *Aspergillus* conidiophore. Courtesy of Dr Hani Zakhour.

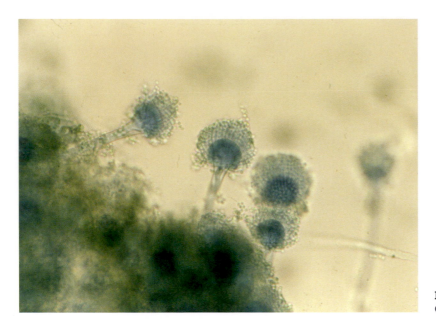

FIGURE 6.19 *Aspergillus* hyphae – high power. Courtesy of Dr Hani Zakhour.

6 months, and every 3 months thereafter. Antibody levels fall slowly. The IgM antibodies disappear first, then the IgA but the IgG antibodies remain positive for years. It has been suggested that after 3 years, treatment can be stopped if the level of IgG against phase-I antigens is still below 400 and IgA against phase-I are no longer detectable [117].

For *Brucella* endocarditis, consultation with a microbiologist is essential and culture bottles may need to be kept for up to 6 weeks. The combination of doxycycline (100 mg twice daily) and IV gentamicin for 4 weeks followed by the combination of doxycycline and rifampicin (600 mg twice daily) for 4–8 weeks is the most effective regimen [118]. Most require valve replacement in combination with antimicrobial agents given over a prolonged period.

In culture-negative endocarditis, all material excised during cardiac surgery in patients with active IE should be cultured and examined [119].

TREATMENT OF INFECTIVE ENDOCARDITIS IN SPECIFIC CLINICAL SITUATIONS

Intravenous Drug Abuse

Infective endocarditis is one of the most severe complications in IV drug abusers and IV drug addiction one of the most important causes of IE in some urban medical centers [120,121] (Figures 6.20 and 6.21). Infected needle punctures and thrombophlebitis may be evident on the arms or legs of the addicts (Figure 6.22) and subcutaneous

abscesses may also develop and require incision and drainage. Infected deep venous thrombosis in the thigh is another complication of using infected needles (Figure 6.23). Infected carious teeth are an important source of microorganisms which are transferred to drug users' needles by their habit of licking the needles before injecting the drug intravenously (Figure 6.24).

Methicillin-sensitive *S. aureus* is the causative organism in 60–70% of cases, streptococci and enterococci in 15–20%, *P. aeruginosa, Serratia marcescens* and other Gram-negative bacilli in <10%, and *Candida* spp. in <2%; 5% of cases are polymicrobial and 5–10% of cases are culture-negative. The tricuspid valve is most frequently affected (>70%), followed by left-sided valves. Pulmonary valve infection is rare (<1%).

The type of antimicrobial therapy and mode of administration necessary is dependent on the organism(s) responsible, which may be suggested by the type of drug and solvent used by the addict [122–124].

The prognosis of right-sided IE is favorable and in those with uncomplicated native valve IE caused by methicillin-sensitive *S. aureus*, 2 weeks' treatment with IV flucloxacillin plus IV gentamicin may cure the infection [125]. However, once the causative organism has been isolated, therapy has to be adjusted. A standard 4–6 week treatment regimen should be used where there is a slow clinical or microbiological response to antibiotic therapy, right-sided endocarditis complicated by right heart failure, large (>20 mm) valve vegetations, acute respiratory failure, septic metastatic foci outside the lungs or extracardiac complications such as acute renal failure, associated severe

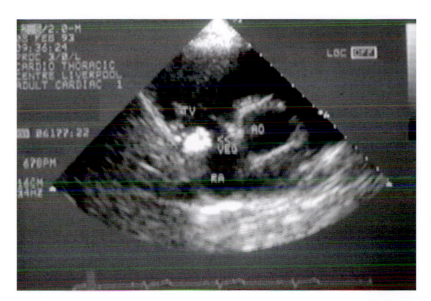

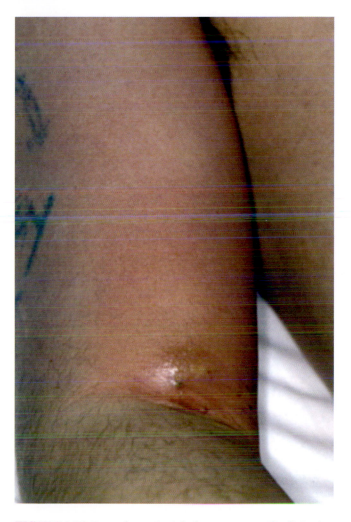

FIGURE 6.20 A 2-D transthoracic echocardiogram showing large vegetation (≪VEG) on the tricuspid valve (TV) in an IV drug abuser with *Staphylococcus aureus* endocarditis. Septic pulmonary infarcts may occur as a result of embolization (AO, aorta; RA, right atrium). Courtesy of Dr Lindsay Morrison.

immunosuppression with or without AIDS, and therapy with antibiotics other than penicillinase-resistant penicillins. It has been estimated that the prevalence of HIV-1 infection in IV drug abusers with endocarditis ranges from 40 to 90% – an important consideration for nursing, medical, surgical, and technical staff [126,127].

Surgery is necessary in <2% of cases and death occurs in <5% of cases. The indications for surgery and the perioperative treatment is the same as in non-addicts but should be more conservative because of the higher incidence of recurrent IE due to continued IV drug abuse. The indication and type of surgery should therefore be carefully

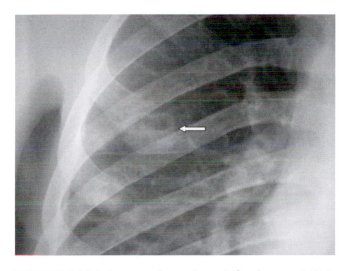

FIGURE 6.21 Pulmonary abscess (arrow) showing a typical air and fluid level, in a 26-year-old IV drug abuser with tricuspid valve endocarditis.

FIGURE 6.22 Large abscess in right forearm as a result of injecting infected drug solution. Courtesy of Dr. N. Beeching.

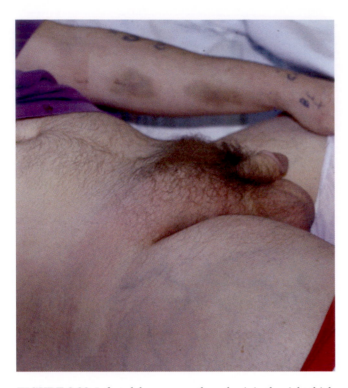

FIGURE 6.23 Infected deep venous thrombosis in the right thigh as a result of injecting infected drug solution into right femoral vein. Infected needle injection sites and thrombophlebitis in the left arm can also be seen. Courtesy of Dr. N. Beeching.

considered to avoid the development of prosthetic valve endocarditis if drug abuse continues. The three main surgical indications are IE due to organisms that are difficult to eradicate, e.g. fungi, persisting bacteremia (>1 week)

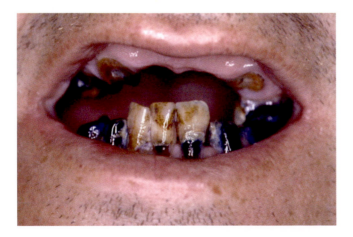

FIGURE 6.24 Infected carious teeth in a drug addict. The practice of licking the needle before injecting IV drugs ensures bacteremia with a mixture of bacteria and the associated risk of infective endocarditis. Courtesy of Dr. N. Beeching.

despite adequate antimicrobial therapy, and large tricuspid valve vegetations (>20 mm) associated with recurrent pulmonary emboli with or without concomitant right heart failure.

HIV-positive Patients

Endocarditis in HIV-positive patients usually occurs as a result of IV drug abuse or long-term indwelling catheters [128]. Estimates of endocarditis occurrence vary from 6.3% to 34% [129]. *S. aureus* is the most frequent causative organism and for drug abusers the tricuspid valve is most commonly affected and short courses of antibiotics have been reported to be successful [130]. Fungal endocarditis is not uncommon and there is an increased risk of *Salmonella* infection [131]. The outcome is worst in patients with AIDS and prolonged IV antibiotics are probably indicated [132–134].

Pregnancy

Most of the first choice antibiotics are safe and effective in pregnancy. Penicillins do not appear to cause maternal or fetal complications [135]. Aminoglycosides should be used only in special situations because of the potential for oto- and nephrotoxicity in the fetus [136]. No teratogenic effects have so far been reported with imipenem or rifampicin. Quinolones are contraindicated in pregnancy [136].

Amphotericin B does not appear to be associated with teratogenic effects, unlike fluconazole where there appears to be a dose-dependent effect [137]. For IE in pregnancy, the advice of an expert microbiologist is strongly advised.

Cardiac surgery for IE in pregnancy is difficult. There is a risk of fetal distress, growth retardation, and fetal death and wherever possible, surgical intervention should be postponed until the fetus is viable and heart surgery and cesarean section can be performed as a concomitant procedure. Close cooperation between cardiologist, cardiac surgeon, and obstetrician is essential. There does not appear to be any absolute indication for pregnancy termination in active IE since in patients with heart failure due to valve insufficiency, hemodynamic improvement cannot be expected by termination of pregnancy alone.

Prosthetic Valve Endocarditis

In early prosthetic valve endocarditis (PVE), *S. epidermidis* and *S. aureus* are the most frequent organisms responsible. Vegetations are generally larger than those found in NVE and prosthetic material protects organisms against antimicrobial treatment – making sterilization with antibiotics extremely difficult [138,139]. Consequently, antibiotics have to be used in dosages that result in maximum but nontoxic serum concentrations in order to penetrate the vegetations, and the duration of treatment must also be longer. Antibiotic sterilization of large vegetations is unlikely with organisms that have a high MIC. A minimum of 2 months' IV therapy may cure some cases [140] but most will require further valve surgery and another month's IV treatment. Beyond 6 months, the organisms causing "late" PVE are not dissimilar to those responsible for NVE [141]. When PVE is clinically apparent and blood cultures are not yet positive, empiric treatment should be initiated with IV vancomycin and gentamicin.

Prosthetic valve endocarditis has a poor prognosis and demands prompt and careful assessment of the need for early surgical intervention [140–147] (Figure 6.25). Transesophageal echocardiography is essential in order to recognize the presence of vegetations on the prosthesis and for diagnosing periprosthetic abscess formation, fistulas, and prosthetic valve dysfunction not seen on a transthoracic study.

In patients with PVE due to aggressive organisms such as *S. aureus*, those who fail to respond immediately to

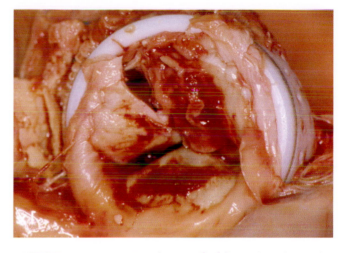

FIGURE 6.25 Destruction of aortic valve bioprosthesis by *Staphylococcus aureus*.

antibiotics, those with large periprosthetic leaks or abscesses, fistula formation and false aneurysms, vegetations on the prosthesis, new-onset conduction disturbance,

TABLE 6.8 Treatment for native valve endocarditis caused by streptococci, enterococci and HACEK organisms: UK, Europe, and USA

Organism	UK	Europe	USA
Penicillin-sensitive viridans streptococci or *S. bovis*	**Benzylpenicillin** 1–2 g IV 4-hourly 4 weeks + **gentamicin** 3–5 mg/kg IV/24 h 2 weeks or **ceftriaxone** 2 g/day IV 4 weeks	**Penicillin G** 2–3 MU IV 4-hourly 4 weeks + **gentamicin** 3 mg/kg IV/24 h 2 weeks or **ceftriaxone** 2 g/day IV 4 weeks	**Penicillin G** 2–3 MU IV 4-hourly 4 weeks or **ceftriaxone** 2 g/day IV 4 weeks
Penicillin-resistant viridans streptococci and *S. bovis*	**Benzylpenicillin** 1–2 g IV 4-hourly 6 weeks + **gentamicin** 3–5 mg/kg IV/24 h 2–4 weeks	**Penicillin G** 3–4 MU IV 4-hourly 4 weeks + **gentamicin** 3 mg/kg IV/24 h in 2–3 doses	**Penicillin G** 3 MU IV 4-hourly 4 weeks + **gentamicin** 1 mg/kg IV/IM 8-hourly 2 weeks
Enterococcus	**Ampicillin** or **amoxicillin** 2 g IV 4-hourly 4–6 weeks + **gentamicin** 3–5 mg/kg IV/24 h 4–6 weeks	**Penicillin G** 3–4 MU IV 4-hourly 4 weeks + **gentamicin** 1.5 mg/kg IV 12-hourly 4 weeks	**Penicillin G** 3–5 MU IV 4-hourly 4–6 weeks or **ampicillin** 2 g IV 4-hourly 4–6 weeks + **gentamicin** 1 mg/kg IV/IM 8-hourly 4–6 weeks
Penicillin allergic individuals	**Vancomycin** 30 mg/kg IV/day in 2 divided doses 4–6 weeks + **gentamicin** 3–5 mg/kg IV/day in 2–3 divided doses 2–6 weeks	**Vancomycin** 30 mg/kg IV/day in 2 divided doses 4–6 weeks ± **gentamicin** 3 mg/kg IV/day in 2 doses 4 weeks	**Vancomycin** 30 mg/kg IV/day in 2 divided doses 4–6 weeks ± **gentamicin** 1 mg/kg IV/IM 8-hourly 4–6 weeks
HACEK group	**Ampicillin** or **amoxicillin** 12 g IV/24 hrs in 4 divided doses 4–6 weeks + **gentamicin** 3–5 mg/kg IV/24 hours 2 weeks or **ceftriaxone** 2 g/day IV 3–4 weeks	**Ceftriaxone** 2 g/day IV 3–4 weeks or **ampicillin** 2 g IV 6-hourly 3–4 weeks + **gentamicin** 1 mg/kg IV 8-hourly 3–4weeks	**Ceftriaxone** 2 g/day IV/IM 4 weeks or **ampicillin** 2 g IV 4-hourly 4 weeks + **gentamicin** 1 mg/kg IV/IM 8-hourly 4 weeks

TABLE 6.9 Treatment for native and prosthetic valve staphylococcal endocarditis: UK, Europe, and USA

	UK	*Europe*	*USA*
Native			
Penicillin-sensitive staphylococci	**Benzylpenicillin** 1.2 g IV 4-hourly 6 weeks + **gentamicin** 3–5 mg/kg IV/day 1 week		
Methicillin-sensitive staphylococci	**Flucloxacillin** 2 g IV 4-hourly 6 weeks + **gentamicin** 3–5 mg/kg IV/day 1 week	**Oxacillin** 2–3 g 6-hourly 4 weeks + **gentamicin** 3 mg/kg IV/day in 3 doses 3–5 days	**Oxacillin** 2 g IV 4-hourly 4–6 weeks + **gentamicin** 1 mg/kg IM/IV 8-hourly 3–5 days
Methicillin-resistant staphylococci or penicillin allergic individuals	**Vancomycin** 30 mg/kg/day IV over 2 h in 2 divided doses 6 weeks + **gentamicin** 3–5 mg/kg IV/day in 3 divided doses 1 week	**Vancomycin** 30 mg/kg/day IV over 2 h in divided doses 6 weeks	**Vancomycin** 30 mg/kg/day IV in 2 divided doses 4–6 weeks
Prosthetic			
Methicillin-sensitive staphylococci	**Flucloxacillin** 2 g IV 4-hourly 6 weeks + **rifampicin** 300 mg orally 8-hourly 6 weeks + **gentamicin** 3–5 mg/kg IV/day in 3 divided doses 2 weeks	**Oxacillin** 2–3 g 6-hourly 6–8 weeks + **rifampicin** 300 mg IV 8-hourly 6–8 weeks + **gentamicin** 3 mg/kg IV/day in 3 divided doses 2 weeks	**Oxacillin** 2 g IV 4-hourly 6–8 weeks + **rifampicin** 300 mg orally 8-hourly 6–8 weeks + **gentamicin** 3 mg/kg IV/day in 3 divided doses 2 weeks
Methicillin-resistant	**Vancomycin** 30 mg/kg IV/day in 2 divided doses over 2 h for 6 weeks + **rifampicin** 300 mg orally 8-hourly 6 weeks + **gentamicin** 3–5 mg/kg IV/day in 3 divided doses 2 weeks	**Vancomycin** 30 mg/kg IV/day in 2 divided doses over 2 h for 6 weeks + **rifampicin** 300 mg IV/day in 3 divided doses 6–8 weeks + **gentamicin** 3 mg/kg IV/day in 3 divided doses 6–8 weeks	**Vancomycin** 30 mg/kg IV/day in 2 divided doses over 2 h for 6–8 weeks + **rifampicin** 300 mg orally 8-hourly 6–8 weeks + **gentamicin** 3 mg/kg IV/day in 3 divided doses 2 weeks

heart failure due to prosthetic valve dysfunction and fungal infection require surgery urgently [148–153]. It is a forlorn hope that these situations will be cured by medical treatment alone as surgical mortality is probably related to the amount of anatomical destruction that has already occurred.

Although, superior results have been shown with surgical treatment compared with antibiotics alone, occasionally medical treatment alone may be appropriate [140,154–160]. Patients in whom the diagnosis is made early, those with streptococcal infection, a prompt antibiotic response, favorable transesophageal echocardiographic findings such as small or absent vegetations, and no periprosthetic abscesses or prosthetic dysfunction may be managed conservatively. However, they require careful clinical monitoring and should be reconsidered for surgery if complications arise – as happens not infrequently [140,158]. Patients in whom surgery is contraindicated

for some other reason or who refuse to give consent for surgery may also be managed medically. Mortality, however, is significant (26–70%) [161,162].

A comparison between the treatment regimens recommended in the UK, Europe, and the USA is shown in Tables 6.8 and 6.9.

PENICILLIN ALLERGY

Patients with a *convincing* history of immediate-type (IgE-mediated) hypersensitivity reaction to penicillin including urticarial rash or angioneurotic edema should not receive penicillin, cephalosporin or other B-lactam antibiotics (Figures 6.26 and 6.27). Vancomycin or teicoplanin should be substituted and given with gentamicin, although the risk of nephrotoxicity increases and requires careful monitoring.

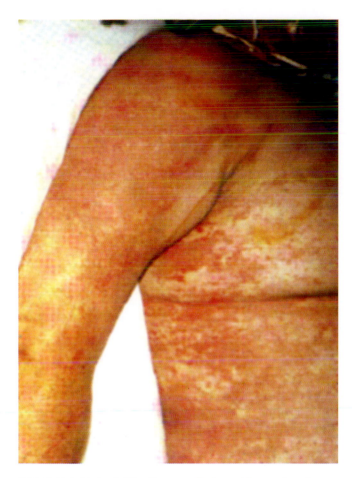

FIGURE 6.26 Penicillin allergy results in a widespread erythematous maculopapular rash and when severe may result in a recurrence of pyrexia.

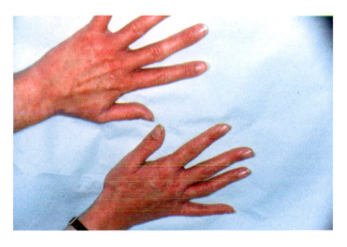

FIGURE 6.27 Penicillin hypersensitivity rash on hands. Courtesy of Dr Graham Sharpe.

ANTICOAGULANT THERAPY

For patients on long-term oral anticoagulants (e.g. for mechanical valve prosthesis), coumarin therapy should be discontinued and replaced by heparin immediately after the diagnosis of IE is confirmed.

MONITORING OF PLASMA DRUG LEVELS

Most treatment regimens require regular monitoring of plasma antimicrobial concentrations. Peak and trough levels should be checked twice weekly, but more frequently in the elderly and in those with renal or hepatic impairment in order to minimize the risk of toxicity (e.g. with aminoglycosides or glycopeptides) and to ensure that bactericidal concentrations are maintained [2,163]. Monitoring of drug levels will generally require close liaison with the microbiologist. For vancomycin, trough levels between 10 and 15 mg/L would be considered efficient. For teicoplanin (generally not recommended for treatment of IE due to *S. aureus*) a peak level >20 mg/L may be optimum in Grampositive endocarditis and a trough level >20 mg/L may be as effective as vancomycin in the treatment of *S. aureus* endocarditis [164,165].

In those patients with impaired renal function, the starting dose of most antibiotics should be modified and thereafter serum levels should be monitored closely and the dose and/or frequency of administration adjusted accordingly. This applies to penicillin, ampicillin, and amoxicillin as well as teicoplanin, gentamicin, and vancomycin.

RESPONSE TO TREATMENT

Patients should be monitored frequently to assess the response to treatment, to detect complications promptly, and to reappraise the need for surgical intervention. Assessment should include clinical examination, measurement of body temperature, ECG, blood count, ESR and CRP, renal and hepatic function tests, and repeat echocardiograms.

Most patients improve during the first week of effective antimicrobial therapy and the temperature should normalize within 5–10 days. CRP values usually decrease rapidly during the first or second week but may remain slightly elevated for 4–6 weeks. A persistently elevated CRP suggests inadequately controlled infection with cardiac or septic complications. ESR is less useful for reflecting the therapeutic response, since high values may persist over several weeks despite clinical improvement. Persistence or recurrence of fever may not only be due to inadequate

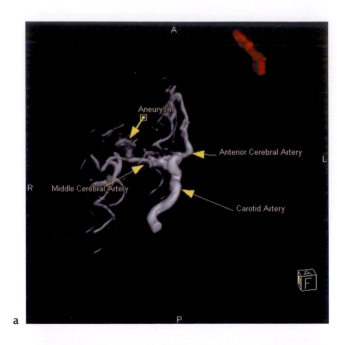

a

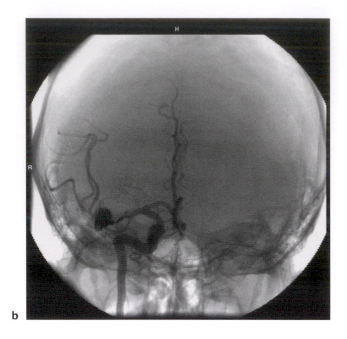

b

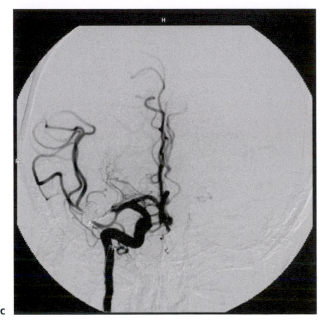

c

FIGURE 6.28 (a) 3D reconstruction of right carotid angiogram showing a large mycotic aneurysm of the right middle cerebral artery in a 63-year-old marine engineer with severe aortic and mitral regurgitation due to *Enterococcus faecalis* infective endocarditis. Four weeks into treatment with IV amoxicillin and gentamicin he developed severe headache and neck stiffness due to subarachnoid haemorrhage. Although he had no neurological deficit, CAT digital subtraction angiography showed a large right middle cerebral artery aneurysm. (b and c) The aneurysm was successfully occluded by intravascular coil placement prior to aortic and mitral valve replacement. Courtesy of Dr. N Newall and Dr. S Niven.

therapy but to myocardial or metastatic abscesses, recurrent emboli, venous thrombosis extending from the site of venous cannulation, superinfection, or febrile reaction to the antibiotics (commonly recurrence of fever) [166]. Persisting bacteremia indicates persisting infection as does persisting leukocytosis.

If a rash develops, the antibiotics should be changed unless the antimicrobial therapy options are very limited.

Weight gain, improvement of appetite, and a rise in hemoglobin may not occur for weeks after treatment and

splenomegaly takes months to resolve. New or changing heart murmurs due to valvular destruction may occur during or after therapy and must be sought by regular physical examination during the period of treatment. Heart failure may develop and is the principal cause of death, especially in aortic valve endocarditis. The natural history of vegetations during successful medical treatment of IE has been described by Vuille et al [167]. Echocardiography should be performed at any time during the course of treatment if the symptoms or physical signs change and at the end

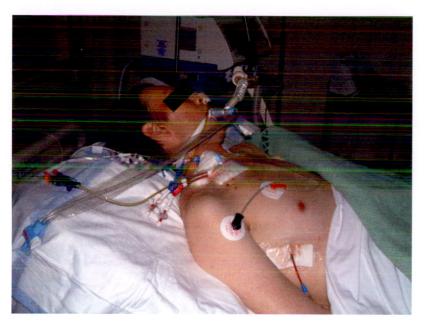

FIGURE 6.29 Thirty-year-old IV drug abuser after aortic valve replacement for severe infective endocarditis due to *Staphylococcus aureus*. He suffered acute renal failure requiring hemofiltration via the right subclavian artery and vein as well as bowel infarction and peritonitis requiring bowel resection. Courtesy of Dr Nigel Scawn.

of treatment to document the site and extent of valvular damage and as a baseline for long-term follow-up.

Mycotic aneurysms may regress on antimicrobial therapy or rupture weeks or years later. Central nervous system symptoms/physical signs suggest cerebral aneurysm formation with leakage or enlargement and demand urgent investigation by CAT/MRI scanning and treatment (Figure 6.28).

Renal insufficiency from glomerulonephritis usually improves with treatment, but not always, and a specialist opinion should be sought early. Other causes of renal insufficiency include hemodynamic instability, antibiotic drug toxicity, renal infarction and systemic embolization, and contrast media toxicity; or it may be a postoperative phenomenon. Hemofiltration or dialysis may be required (Figures 6.29 and 6.30).

RELAPSE/NEW EPISODES

If a primary focus responsible for IE is identified, it should be eliminated prior to an elective cardiac surgical

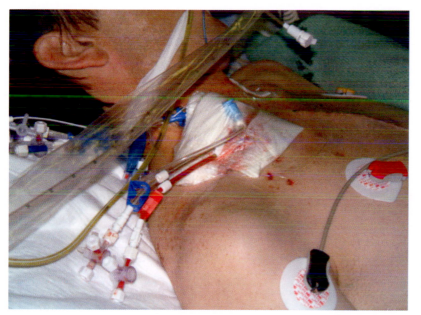

FIGURE 6.30 Close-up view of arterial and venous hemofiltration lines placed into the right subclavian artery and vein via a supraclavicular approach. Courtesy of Dr Nigel Scawn.

procedure in an attempt to prevent relapse. Following medical or surgical treatment of IE, all patients require careful follow-up for signs of clinical relapse or hemodynamic deterioration [168]. Most relapses occur within 2 months of stopping treatment and most within 4 weeks. The reported relapse rate is <2% for streptococcal IE in native valves, but is considerably higher for virulent organisms such as staphylococci and enterococci (8–20%) and for PVE (10–15%). Difficult-to-treat organisms such as *Brucella*,*Chlamydia*, and *Bartonella*, and polymicrobial IE seen in IV drug abusers, are associated with an increased relapse rate, as are a suboptimal choice of antibiotic therapy or insufficient duration of treatment. Blood cultures 2–4 weeks after completion of treatment detect most relapses. Delayed relapses may occur with fungal and Q-fever endocarditis. When relapse occurs in patients with PVE after a course of medical therapy, a perivalvular infection is usually present and further surgery is usually required.

New episodes may occur in 6% of patients with NVE although IV drug abusers are more susceptible [169].

OUTPATIENT TREATMENT

Because of the high morbidity and mortality associated with IE and the need for continued clinical observation and investigations to monitor progress and response to treatment, inpatient management is essential and only in exceptional circumstances would outpatient treatment be considered acceptable – and only then, after an initial period of hospitalization and stabilization [170,171].

REFERENCES

1. Besnier JM, Choutet P. Medical treatment of infective endocarditis: general principles. Eur Heart J 1995;16(Suppl B):72–74.
2. Leport C, Horstkotte D, Burckhardt D and the Group of Experts of the International Society for Chemotherapy. Antibiotic prophylaxis for infective endocarditis from an international group of experts towards a European consensus. Eur Heart J 1995;16(Suppl B):126–131.
3. Working Party of the British Society for Antimicrobial Chemotherapy. Antibiotic treatment of streptococcal, enterococcal and staphylococcal endocarditis. Guidelines. Heart 1998;79:207–210.
4. Bayer AS, Bolger AF, Taubert KA, et al. Diagnosis and management of infective endocarditis and its complications. Circulation 1998;98:2936–2948.
5. The Task Force on Infective Endocarditis of the European Society of Cardiology. Guidelines on Prevention, Diagnosis and Treatment of Infective Endocarditis. Executive Summary. Eur Heart J 2004;25:267–276.
6. Advisory Group of the British Cardiac Society Clinical Practice Committee and the Royal College of Physicians Clinical Effectiveness and Evaluation Unit. The Prophylaxis and Treatment of Infective Endocarditis in Adults. www.bcs.com.
7. Wilson W, Karchmer A, Dajani A, et al. Antibiotic treatment of adults with infective endocarditis due to streptococci, enterococci, staphylococci and HACEK microorganisms. JAMA 1995;274:1706–1713.
8. ACC/AHA guidelines for the management of patients with valvular heart disease. A report of the American College of Cardiology/American Heart Association. Task force on practice guidelines (Committee on Management of Patients with Valvular Heart Disease). J Am Coll Cardiol 1998;32:1486–1588.
9. Scheld WM. Pathogenesis and pathophysiology of infective endocarditis. In: Sande MA, Kaye D, Root RK, eds. Endocarditis. New York: Churchill Livingstone; 1984:1–32.
10. Durack DT, Beeson PB. Experimental bacterial endocarditis. II. Survival of bacteria in endocardial vegetations. Br J Exp Pathol 1972;53:50–53.
11. Washington JA. In vitro testing of antimicrobial agents. Infect Dis Clin North Am 1989;3:375–387.
12. Mulligan MJ, Cobbs CG. Bacteriostatic versus bactericidal activity. Infect Dis Clin North Am 1989;3:389–398.
13. Holloway Y, Dankert J, Hess J. Penicillin tolerance and bacterial endocarditis. Lancet 1980;i:589.
14. Eliopoulos GM. Synergism and antagonism. Infect Dis Clin North Am 1989;3:399–406.
15. Watanakunakorn C, Glotzbecker C. Synergism with aminoglycosides of penicillin, ampicillin and vancomycin against nonenterococcal group-D streptococci and viridans streptococci. J Med Microbiol 1976;10:133–138.
16. Sande MA, Irvin RG. Penicillin-aminoglycoside synergy in experimental *Streptococcus viridans* endocarditis. J Infect Dis 1974;129:572–576.
17. Mandell GL, Kaye D, Levison ME, Hook EW. Enterococcal endocarditis: an analysis of 38 patients observed at the New York Hospital-Cornell Medical Center. Arch Intern Med 1970;125:258–264.
18. Bisno AL, Dismukes WE, Durack DT, et al. Antimicrobial treatment of infective endocarditis due to viridans streptococci, enterococci and staphylococci. JAMA 1989;261:1471–1477.
19. Moellering RC. Treatment of enterococcal endocarditis. In: Sande MA, Kaye D, Root RK, eds. Endocarditis. New York: Churchill Livingstone; 1984:113–133.
20. Wilson WR, Geraci JE. Treatment of streptococcal infective endocarditis. Am J Med 1985;78(Suppl 6B):128–137.
21. Gutschik E and the Endocarditis Working Group of the International Society of Chemotherapy. Microbiological recommendations for the diagnosis and follow-up of infective endocarditis. Clin Microbiol Infect 1998;4(Suppl 3):S10–16.

22. Weinstein MP, Stratton CW, Ackley A, et al. Multicenter collaborative evaluation of a standardized serum bactericidal test as a prognostic indicator in infective endocarditis. Am J Med 1985;78:262–269.

23. MacMahon SW, Roberts JK, Kramer-Fox R, et al. Mitral valve prolapse and infective endocarditis. Am Heart J 1987;113:1291–1298.

24. Facklam RR, Carey RB. Streptococci and aerococci. In: Lennete EH, Balows A, Hausler WJ Jr, et al, eds. Manual of Clinical Microbiology, 4th edn. Washington, DC: American Society of Microbiology; 1985:154–175.

25. Karchmer AW. Staphylococcal endocarditis. Laboratory and clinical basis for antibiotic therapy. Am J Med 1985;78(Suppl 6B):116–127.

26. Eykyn SJ. Staphylococcal sepsis. The changing pattern of disease and therapy. Lancet 1988;i:100–104.

27. Chambers HF, Korzeniowski OM, Sande MA. *Staphylococcus aureus* endocarditis: clinical manifestations in addicts and non-addicts. Medicine 1983;62:170–177.

28. McKinsey DS, Ratts TE, Bisno AL. Underlying cardiac lesions in adults with infective endocarditis: the changing spectrum. Am J Med 1987;82:681–688.

29. Espersen F, Frimodt-Moller N. *Staphylococcus aureus* endocarditis. A review of 119 cases. Arch Intern Med 1986;146:1118–1121.

30. Terpenning MS, Buggy BP, Kauffman CA. Infective endocarditis: clinical features in young and elderly patients. Am J Med 1987;83:626–634.

31. Caputo GM, Archer GL, Calderwood SB, et al. Native valve endocarditis due to coagulase-negative staphylococci. Clinical and microbiologic features. Am J Med 1987;83:619–625.

32. Francioli P. Antibiotic treatment of streptococcal and enterococcal endocarditis: an overview. Eur Heart J 1995;16(Suppl B):75–79.

33. Bille J. Medical treatment of staphylococcal infective endocarditis. Eur Heart J 1995;16(Suppl B):80–83.

34. Korzeniowski O, Sande MA. Combination antimicrobial therapy for *Staphylococcus aureus* endocarditis in patients addicted to parenteral drugs and in non-addicts. A prospective study. Ann Intern Med 1982;97:496–503.

35. Besnier JM, Leport C, Bure A, Vilde JL. Vancomycin-aminoglycoside combinations in therapy of endocarditis caused by *Enterococcus* species and *Streptococcus bovis*. Eur J Clin Microbiol Infect Dis 1990;9:130–133.

36. Pollock AA, Tee PE, Patel IH, et al. Pharmacokinetic characteristics of IV ceftriaxone in normal adults. Antimicrob Agents Chemother 1981;22:816–823.

37. Francioli P, Etienne J, Hoigne R, et al. Treatment of streptococcal endocarditis with a single daily dose of devtriaxone sodium for 4 weeks. Efficacy and out-patient treatment feasibility. JAMA 1992;267:264–267.

38. Johnson AP, Warner M, Broughton K, et al. Antibiotic susceptibility of streptococci and related genera causing endocarditis: analysis of UK reference laboratory referrals, January 1996–March 2000. Br Med J 2001;322:395–396.

39. Sexton DJ, Tenenbaum MJ, Wilson WR, et al. Ceftriaxone once daily for four weeks compared with ceftriaxone plus gentamicin once daily for two weeks for treatment of endocarditis due to penicillin-susceptible streptococci. Endocarditis Treatment Consortium Group. Clin Infect Dis 1998;27:1470–1474.

40. Wilson WR. Ceftriaxone sodium therapy of penicillin G-susceptible streptococcal endocarditis. JAMA 1992;267:279–280.

41. Garcia Rodriguez JF, Mesias Prego JA, Dominguez Gomez D. Treatment of endocarditis due to penicillin-susceptible streptococci with a two-week course of ceftriaxone followed by oral amoxicillin. Eur J Clin Microbiol Infect Dis 1992;11:952–953.

42. Francioli P, Ruch W, Stamboulian D. Treatment of streptococcal endocarditis with a single daily dose of ceftriaxone and netilmicin for 14 days: a prospective multicenter study. Clin Infect Dis 1995;21:1406–1410.

43. Myers JP, Linnemann CC Jr. Bacteremia due to methicillin-resistant *Staphylococcus aureus*. J Infect Dis 1982; 145:532–536.

44. Archer AW. Antibiotic therapy of nonenterococcal streptococcal and staphylococcal endocarditis: current regimens and some future considerations. J Antimicrob Chemother 1988;21(Suppl C):91–106.

45. Karchmer AW, Archer GL, Dismukes WE. *Staphylococcus epidermidis* causing prosthetic valve endocarditis: microbiologic and clinical observations as guides to therapy. Ann Intern Med 1983;98:447–455.

46. Heimberger TS, Duma RJ. Infection of prosthetic heart valves and cardiac pacemakers. Infect Dis Clin North Am 1989;3:221–245.

47. Faville RJ Jr, Zaske DE, Kaplan EL, et al. *Staphylococcus aureus* endocarditis: combined therapy with vancomycin and rifampicin. JAMA 1978;240:1963–1965.

48. Acar JF, Goldstein FW, Duval J. Use of rifampicin for the treatment of serious staphylococcal and gram-negative bacillary infections. Rev Infect Dis 1983;5:(Suppl 3)502–506.

49. Linares J. The VISA/GISA problem: therapeutic implications. Clin Microbiol Infect 2001;7(Suppl 4):8–15.

50. Dehondt G, Leven M, Vandermersch C, Colaert J. Destructive endocarditis caused by *Staphylococcus lugdunensis*: case report and review of the literature. Acta Clin Belg 1997;52:27–30.

51. Vandenesch F, Etienne J, Reverdy ME, Eykyn SJ. Endocarditis due to *Staphylococcus lugdunensis*: report of 11 cases and review. Clin Infect Dis 1993;17:871–876.

52. Lessing MP, Crook DW, Bowler IC, Gribbin B. Native valve endocarditis caused by *Staphylococcus lugdunensis*. QJM 1996;89:855–858.

53. Roberts RB, Kriger AG, Schiller NL, Gross KC. Viridans streptococcal endocarditis: role of various species, including pyridoxal-dependent streptococci. Rev Infect Dis 1979;1:955–965.

54. Stein DS, Nelson KE. Endocarditis due to nutritionally deficient streptococci: therapeutic dilemma. Rev Infect Dis 1987;9:908–916.

55. Bouvet A. Human endocarditis due to nutritionally variant streptococci: *Streptococcus adjacens* and *Streptococcus defectivus*. Eur Heart J 1995;16(Suppl B):24–27.

56. Hricak V Jr, Kovacik J, Marx P, et al. Endocarditis due to *Enterococcus faecalis*: risk factors and outcome in 21 cases from a 5 year National Survey. Scand J Infect Dis 1998;30:540–541.

57. Johnson AP, Warner M, Woodford N, et al. Antibiotic resistance among enterococci causing endocarditis in the UK: analysis of isolates referred to a reference laboratory. Br Med J 1998;317:629–630.

58. Landman D, Quale JM. Management of infections due to resistant enterococci: a review of therapeutic options. J Antimicrob Chemother 1997;40:161–170.

59. Antony SJ, Ladner J, Stratton CW, et al. High-level aminoglycoside-resistant enterococcus causing endocarditis successfully treated with a combination of ampicillin, imipenem and vancomycin. Scand J Infect Dis 1997;29:628–630.

60. Lee PY, Das SS. Endocarditis due to high-level gentamicin-resistant *Enterococcus faecalis*. Postgrad Med J 1995;71:117–119.

61. Matsumura S, Simor AE. Treatment of endocarditis due to vancomycin-resistant *Enterococcus faecium* with quinupristin/dalfopristin, doxycycline, and rifampicin: a synergistic drug combination. Clin Infect Dis 1998;27:1554–1556.

62. Brisk AJ, van der Ende J, Routier RJ, Devenish L. A case of vancomycin-resistant enterococcal endocarditis. S Afr Med J 2000;90:1113–1115.

63. Zervos MJ, Terpenning MS, Schaberg DR, et al. High-level aminoglycoside-resistant enterococci. Colonization of nursing home and acute care hospital patients. Arch Intern Med 1987;147:1591–1594.

64. Wilson WR, Wilkowske CJ, Wright AJ, et al. Treatment of streptomycin-susceptible and streptomycin-resistant enterococcal endocarditis. Ann Intern Med 1984;100:816–823.

65. Hood S, Baxter RH. *Listeria* endocarditis causing aortic root abscess and fistula to the left atrium. Scott Med J 1999;44:117–118.

66. Moreira AL, Haslett PA, Symmons WF. *Proprionibacterium acnes* as the cause of endocarditis in a liver transplant recipient. Clin Infect Dis 2000;30:224–226.

67. Mitchell AR, Hayak LJ. *Lactobacillus* endocarditis. J Infect 1999;38:200–201.

68. Huynh TT, Walling AD, Miller MA, et al. *Proprionibacterium acnes* endocarditis. Can J Cardiol 1995;11:785–787.

69. Morrison DJ, Sperling LS, Schwartz DA, Felmer JM. *Escherichia coli* endocarditis of a native aortic valve. Arch Pathol Lab Med 1997;121:1292–1295.

70. Anderson MJ, Janoff EN. *Klebsiella* endocarditis: report of two cases and review. Clin Infect Dis 1998;26:468–474.

71. Ananthasubramanian K, Karthikeyan V. Aortic ring abscess and aortoatrial fistula complicating fulminant prosthetic valve endocarditis due to *Proteus mirabilis*. J Ultrasound Med 2000;19:63–66.

72. Raymond NJ, Robertson MD, Lang SD. Aortic valve endocarditis due to *Escherichia coli*. Clin Infect Dis 1992;15:749–750.

73. Thomas MG, Rowland-Jones S, Smyth E. *Klebsiella pneumoniae* endocarditis. J R Soc Med 1989;82:114–115.

74. Donowitz GR, Mandell GL. Beta-lactam antibiotics. N Engl J Med 1988;318:419–426.

75. Donowitz GR. Third generation cephalosporins. Infect Dis Clin North Am 1989;3:595–612.

76. Sobel JD. Imipenem and aztreonam. Infect Dis Clin North Am 1989;3:613–624.

77. Lipman B, Neu HC. Imipenem: a new carbapenem antibiotic. Update on antibiotics II. Med Clin North Am 1988;72:567–579.

78. Dickinson G, Rodriguez K, Arcey S, et al. Efficacy of imipenem/cilastatin in endocarditis. Am J Med 1985;78:(6A)117–121.

79. Neu HC. Aztreonam: The first monobactam. Med Clin North Am 1988;72:555–566.

80. Bush LM, Calmon J, Johnson CC. Newer penicillins and beta-lactamase inhibitors. Infect Dis Clin North Am 1989;3:571–594.

81. Reyes MP, Lerner AM. Current problems in the treatment of infective endocarditis due to *Pseudomonas aeruginosa*. Rev Infect Dis 1983;5:314–321.

82. Cohen PS, Maguire JH, Weinstein L. Infective endocarditis caused by gram-negative bacteria: a review of the literature. Prog Cardiovasc Dis 1980;22:205–242.

83. Komshian SV, Tablan OC, Palutke W, Reyes MP. Characteristics of left-sided endocarditis due to *Pseudomonas aeruginosa* in the Detroit Medical Center. Rev Infect Dis 1990;12:693–702.

84. Carvajal A, Frederiksen W. Fatal endocarditis due to *Listeria monocytogenes*. Rev Infect Dis 1988;10:616–623.

85. Lindner PS, Hardy DJ, Murphy TF. Endocarditis due to *Corynebacterium pseudodiphtheriticum*. NY State J Med 1986;86:102–104.

86. Nord CE. Anaerobic bacteria in septicaemia and endocarditis. Scand J Infect Dis 1982;31(Suppl):95–104.

87. Weber G, Borer A, Riesenberg K, Schlaeffer F. Infective endocarditis due to *Fusobacterium nucleatum* in an intravenous drug abuser. Eur J Clin Microbiol Infect Dis 1999;18:655–657.

88. Shammas NW, Murphy GW, Eichelberger J, et al. Infective endocarditis due to *Fusobacterium nucleatum*: case report and review of the literature. Clin Cardiol 1993;16:72–75.

89. Tornos MP, Almirante B, Pahissa A, et al. Prosthetic valve endocarditis caused by gram-negative bacilli of the HACEK group. Am J Med 1990;88(Suppl N):64N.

90. Das M, Badley AD, Cockerill FR, et al. Infective endocarditis caused by HACEK microorganisms. Annu Rev Med 1997;48:25–33.

91. Lesage V, Van Pee D, Luyx C, et al. Septic arthritis caused by *Haemophilus influenzae* associated with endocarditis. Clin Rheumatol 1998;17:340–342.

92. Darras-Joly C, Lortholary O, Mainardi JL, et al. *Haemophilus* endocarditis: report of 42 cases in adults and review. Haemophilus Endocarditis Study Group. Clin Infect Dis 1997;24:1087–1094.

93. Lin BH, Vieco PT. Intracranial mycotic aneurysm in a patient with endocarditis caused by *Cardiobacterium hominis*. Can Assoc Radiol J 1995;46:40–42.

94. Le Quellec A, Bessis D, Perez C, Ciurana AJ. Endocarditis due to beta-lactamase-producing *Cardiobacterium hominis*. Clin Infect Dis 1994;19:994–995.

95. Pritchard TM, Foust RT, Cantely JR, Leman RB. Prosthetic valve endocarditis due to *Cardiobacterium hominis* occurring after gastrointestinal endoscopy. Am J Med 1991;90:516–518.

96. Olopoenia LA, Mody V, Reynolds M. *Eikenella corrodens* endocarditis in an intravenous drug user: case report and literature review. J Natl Med Assoc 1994;86:313–315.

97. Chakraborty RN, Meigh RE, Kaye GC. *Kingella kingae* prosthetic valve endocarditis. Indian Heart J 1999;51:438–439.

98. Hassan IJ, Hayek L. Endocarditis caused by *Kingella denitrificans*. J Infect 1993;27:291–295.

99. Lynn DJ, Kane JG, Parker RH. *Haemophilus parainfluenzae* and *influenzae* endocarditis: a review of 40 cases. Medicine 1977;56:115–128.

100. Ellner JJ, Rosenthal MS, Lerner PI, McHenry MC. Infective endocarditis caused by slow-growing, fastidious, gram-negative bacteria. Medicine 1979;58:145–158.

101. Schack SH, Smith PW, Penn RG, Rapoport JM. Endocarditis caused by *Actinobacillus actinomycetemcomitans*. J Clin Microbiol 1984; 20:579–581.

102. Decker MD, Graham BS, Hunter EB, Liebowitz SM. Endocarditis and infections of intravascular devices due to *Eikenella corrodens*. Am J Med Sci 1986;292:209–212.

103. Jenny DB, Letendre PW, Iverson G. Endocarditis due to *Kingella* species. Rev Infect Dis 1988;10:1065–1066.

104. Rubinstein E, Noriega ER, Simberkoff MS, Holzman R, Rahal Jr JJ. Fungal endocarditis: analysis of 24 cases and review of the literature. Medicine 1975;54:331–344.

105. Donal E, Abgueguen P, Coisne D, et al. Echocardiographic features of *Candida* species endocarditis: 12 cases and a review of published reports. Heart 2001;86:179–182.

106. Woods GL, Wood RP, Shaw BW Jr. *Aspergillus* endocarditis in patients without prior cardiovascular surgery: report of a case in a liver transplant recipient and review. Rev Infect Dis 1989;11:263–272.

107. Johnston PG, Lee J, Domanski M, et al. Late recurrent *Candida* endocarditis. Chest 1991;99:1531–1533.

108. Rubinstein E, Lang R. Fungal endocarditis. Eur Heart J 1995;16(Suppl B):84–89.

109. Ellis M. Fungal endocarditis. J Infect 1997;35:99–103.

110. Muehrcke DD, Lytle BW, Cosgrove DM. Surgical and long-term antifungal therapy for fungal prosthetic valve endocarditis. Ann Thorac Surg 1995;60:538–543.

111. Remsey ES, Lytle BW. Repair of fungal aortic prosthetic valve endocarditis associated with periannular abscess. J Heart Valve Dis 1998;7:235–239.

112. Zedtwitz-Liebenstein K, Gabriel H, Willinger B, et al. Prosthetic valve endocarditis due to *Candida tropicalis* complicated by multiple pseudoaneurysms. Infection 2001;29:177–179.

113. Nasser RM, Melgar GR, Longworth DL, et al. Incidence and risk of developing fungal prosthetic valve endocarditis after nosocomial candidemia. Am J Med 1997;103:25–32.

114. Uddin MJ, Sanyal SC, Mustafa AS, et al. The role of aggressive medical therapy along with early surgical intervention in the cure of *Brucella* endocarditis. Ann Thorac Cardiiovasc Surg 1998;4:209–213.

115. Quiroga J, Miralles A, Farinola T, et al. Surgical treatment of *Brucella* endocarditis. Cardiovasc Surg 1996;4:227–230.

116. Raoult D, Houpikian P, Tissot Dupont H, et al. Treatment of Q-fever endocarditis: comparison of two regimens containing doxycycline and ofloxacin or hydroxychloroquine. Arch Intern Med 1999;159:167–173.

117. Raoult D, Raza A, Marrie TJ. Q fever endocarditis and other forms of chronic Q fever. In: Marrie TJ, ed. Q Fever. Vol. I: The Disease. Boston: CRC Press; 1990:179–199.

118. Madkour MM. Brucellosis. In: Fauci AS, et al, eds. Harrison's Principles of Internal Medicine, 14th edn, vol. I. New York: McGraw Hill 1998: Ch 162.

119. Bruneval P, Choucair J, Paraf F, et al. Detection of fastidious bacteria in cardiac valves in case of blood-culture negative endocarditis. J Clin Pathol 2001;54:238–240.

120. Cerubin CE, Sapira JD. The medical complications of drug addiction and the medical assessment of the IV drug user. Ann Intern Med 1993;119:1017–1028.

121. Haverkos HW, Lange WR. Serious infections other than human immunodeficiency virus among intravenous drug abusers. J Infect Dis 1990;161:894–902.

122. Heldman AW, Hartert TV, Ray SC, et al. Oral antibiotic treatment of right-sided staphylococcal endocarditis in injection drug users: prospective randomized comparison with parenteral therapy. Am J Med 1996;101:68–76.

123. Botsford KB, Weinstein RA, Nathan CR, Kabis SA. Selective survival in pentazocine and tripelennamine of *Pseudomonas aeruginosa* serotype 011 from drug addicts. J Infect Dis 1985;151:209–216.

124. Bisbe J, Miro JM, Latone X, et al. Disseminated candidiasis in addicts who use brown heroin. Report of 83 cases and review. Clin Infect Dis 1992;15:910–923.

125. Fortun J, Novase E, Martinez-Beltran J, et al. Short-course therapy for right-side endocarditis due to *Staphylococcus aureus* in drug abusers: cloxacillin versus glycopeptides in combination with gentamicin. Clin Infect Dis 2001;33:120–125.

126. Ribera E, Miro JM, Cortes E, et al. Influence of human immunodeficiency virus 1 infection and degree of immunosuppression in the clinical characteristics and outcome of infective endocarditis in intravenous drug users. Arch Intern Med 1998;158:2043–2050.

127. Palepu A, Cheung SS, Montessori V, et al. Factors other than the Duke criteria associated with infective endocarditis among injection drug users. Clin Invest Med 2002;25:118–25.

128. Cicalini S, Forcina G, De Rosa FG. Infective endocarditis in patients with human immunodeficiency virus infection. J Infect 2001;42:267–271.

129. Rerkpattanapipat P, Wongpraparut N, Jacobs LE, et al. Cardiac manifestations of acquired immunodeficiency syndrome. Arch Intern Med 2000;160:602–608.

130. DiNubile MJ. Short-course antibiotic therapy for right-sided endocarditis caused by *Staphylococcus aureus* in injection drug users. Ann Intern Med 1994;121:873–876.

131. Fernandez Guerrero ML, Torres Perera R, Gomez Rodrigo J, et al. Infectious endocarditis due to non-typhi Salmonella in patients infected with human immunodeficiency virus: report of two cases and review. Clin Infect Dis 1996;22:853–855.

132. Currie PF, Sutherland GR, Jacob AJ, et al. A review of endocarditis in acquired immunodeficiency syndrome and human immunodeficiency virus infection. Eur Heart J 1985;16(Suppl B):15–18.

133. Kinney EL, Monsuez JJ, Kitzis M, Vittecoq D. Treatment of AIDS-associated heart disease. Angiology 1989;40:970–976.

134. Nahass RG, Weinstein MP, Bartels J, Gocke DJ. Infective endocarditis in intravenous drug users: a comparison of human immunodeficiency virus type 1-negative and -positive patients. J Infect Dis 1990;162:967–970.

135. Heinonen CP, Slone D, Shapiro S. Birth Defects and Drugs in Pregnancy. Littleton, MA: Littleton Publishing Sciences Group; 1977.

136. Dashe JS, Gilstrap LC. Antibiotic use in pregnancy. Obstet Gynecol Clin North Am 1977;24:617–629.

137. King CT, Rogers PD, Cleary JD, Chapman SW. Antifungal therapy during pregnancy. Clin Infect Dis 1998;27:1151–1160.

138. Horstkotte D, Weist K, Rueden H. Better understanding of the pathogenesis of prosthetic valve endocarditis – recent perspectives for prevention strategies. J Heart Valve Dis 1998;7:313–315.

139. Hyde JAJ, Darouiche RO, Costeron JW. Strategies for prophylaxis against prosthetic valve endocarditis. A review article. J Heart Valve Dis 1998;7:316–326.

140. Akowuah EF, Davies W, Oliver S, et al. Prosthetic valve endocarditis: early and late outcome following medical or surgical treatment. Heart 2003;89:269–272.

141. Cowgill LD, Addonizio VP, Hopeman AR, Harken AH. Prosthetic valve endocarditis. Curr Probl Cardiol 1986;11:617–664.

142. Tornos P. Management of prosthetic valve endocarditis: a clinical challenge. Heart 2003;89:245–246.

143. DiSesa VJ, Sloss LJ, Cohn LH. Heart transplantation for intractable prosthetic valve endocarditis. J Heart Transplant 1990;9:142–143.

144. Brottier E, Gin H, Brottier L, et al. Prosthetic valve endocarditis: diagnosis and prognosis. Eur Heart J 1984;5(Suppl C)123–127.

145. Cowgill LD, Addonizio VP, Hopeman AR, Harken AH. A practical approach to prosthetic valve endocarditis. Ann Thorac Surg 1987;43:450–457.

146. Leport C, Vilde JL, Bricaire F, et al. Fifty cases of late prosthetic valve endocarditis: improvement in prognosis over a 15 year period. Br Heart J 1987;58:66–71.

147. Dismukes WE. Prosthetic valve endocarditis. Factors influencing outcome and recommendations for therapy. In: Bisno AL, ed. Treatment of Infective Endocarditis. New York: Grune & Stratton; 1981:167–191.

148. Durack DT. Infective endocarditis. In: Schlant R, Hurst WJ, eds. The Heart, 7th edn companion handbook. New York: McGraw Hill; 1990:153–167.

149. Scheld WM, Sande MA. Endocarditis and intravascular infections. In: Mandell GL, Douglas RG Jr, Dolin R, eds. Principles and Practice of Infectious Diseases, 4th edn. New York: Churchill Livingstone; 1995:740–783.

150. DiNubile MJ, Calderwood SB, Steinhaus DM, Karchmer AW. Cardiac conduction abnormalities complicating native valve active endocarditis. Am J Cardiol 1986;58:1213–1217.

151. Tucker KJ, Johnson JA, Ong T, et al. Medical management of prosthetic aortic valve endocarditis and aortic root abscess. Am Heart J 1993;125:1195–1197.

152. Guzman F, Cartmill I, Holden MP, Freeman R. *Candida* endocarditis: report of four cases. Int J Cardiol 1987;16:131–136.

153. Douglas JL, Cobbs CG. Prosthetic valve endocarditis. In: Kaye D, ed. Infective Endocarditis, 2nd edn. New York: Raven Press; 1992:375–396.

154. Yu VL, Fang GD, Keys TF, et al. Prosthetic valve endocarditis: superiority of surgical valve replacement versus medical therapy only. Ann Thorac Surg 1994;58:1073–1077.

155. Saffle JR, Gardner P, Schoenbaum SC, et al. Prosthetic valve endocarditis: the case for prompt valve replacement. J Thorac Cardiovasc Surg 1977;3:416–420.

156. Lytle BW, Taylor PC, Sapp SK, et al. Surgical treatment of prosthetic valve endocarditis. J Thorac Cardiovasc Surg 1996;111:198–210.

157. Farina G, Vitale N, Piaza L, et al. Long term results of surgery for prosthetic valve endocarditis. J Heart Valve Dis 1994;2:165–171.

158. Moon MR, Miller DL, Moore KA, et al. Treatment of endocarditis with valve replacement: the question of tissue versus mechanical prosthesis. Ann Thorac Surg 2001;71:1164–1171.

159. Trunninger K, Attenhofer CH, Seifert B, et al. Long term follow up of prosthetic valve endocarditis: what characteristics

identify patients who were treated successfully with antibiotics alone. Heart 1999;82:714–720.

160. Karchmer AW, Dismuke WE, Buckley MJ, et al. Late prosthetic valve endocarditis: clinical features influencing therapy. Am J Med 1978;64:199–206.

161. Kuyvenhoven P, Rijk-Zwikkere GL, Hermans J, et al. Prosthetic valve endocarditis: analysis of risk factors for mortality. Eur J Cardiothorac Surg 1994;8:420–424.

162. Ivert TS, Dismukes WE, Cobbs CG, et al. Prosthetic valve endocarditis. Circulation 1984;69:223–232.

163. Chow AW, Azar RM. Glycopeptides and nephrotoxicity. Intensive Care Med 1994;20(Suppl 4):23–29.

164. Leport C, Perronne C, Massip P, et al. Evaluation of teicoplanin for treatment of endocarditis caused by gram-positive cocci in 20 patients. Antimicrob Agents Chemother 1989;33:871–876.

165. Karchmer AW, Bisno AL. Infections of prosthetic heart valves and vascular grafts. In: Bisno AL, Waldvogel F, eds. Infections associated with indwelling medical devices. Washington, DC: ASM; 1989:129–159.

166. Blumberg EA, Robbins N, Adimora A, Lowy FD. Persistent fever in association with infective endocarditis. Clin Infect Dis 1992;15:983–990.

167. Vuille C, Nidorf M, Weyman AE, Picard MH. Natural history of vegetations during successful medical treatment of endocarditis. Am Heart J 1994;128:1200–1209.

168. Mansur AJ, Dal Bo CM, Fukushuma JT, et al. Relapses, recurrence, valve replacement and mortality during the long-term follow-up after infective endocarditis. Am Heart J 2001;141:78–86.

169. Lossos IS, Oren R. Recurrent infective endocarditis. Postgrad Med J 1993;69:816–818.

170. Nathwani D, Conlon C on behalf of the OHPAT Workshop. Outpatient and home parenteral antibiotic therapy (OHPAT) in the UK: a consensus statement by a working party. Clin Microbiol Infect 1998;4:537–551.

171. Fancioli PB, Stamboulian D for the Endocarditis Working Group of the International Society for Chemotherapy. Outpatient treatment of infective endocarditis. Clin Microbiol Infect 1998;4(3):S47–55.

172. Wilson APR, Gaya H. Treatment of endocarditis with teicoplanin: a retrospective analysis of 104 cases. J Antimicrob Chemother 1996;38:507–521.

173. Burkert T, Watanakunakorn C. Group A streptococcus endocarditis: report of five cases and review of literature. J Infect 1991;23:307–316.

174. Plastino KA, Connors JE, Spinler SA. Possible synergy between aminoglycosides and vancomycin in the treatment of *Staphylococcus epidermidis* endocarditis? Ann Pharmacother 1994;28:737–739.

175. Whitby M. Fusidic acid in septicaemia and endocarditis.. Int J Antimicrob Agents 1999;12(Suppl 2):S17–22.

176. Fantin B, Leclerq R, Duval J, Carbon C. Fusidic acid alone or in combination with vancomycin for therapy of experimental endocarditis due to methicillin-resistant *Staphylococcus aureus*. Antimicrob Agents Chemother 1993;37:2466–2469.

177. Eykyn SJ. Staphylococcal bacteraemia and endocarditis and fusidic acid. J Antimicrob Chemother 1990;25(Suppl B):33–38.

178. Fichtenbaum CJ, Smith MJ. Treatment of endocarditis due to *Pseudomonas aeruginosa* with imipenem. Clin Infect Dis 1992;14:353–354.

179. Sailler L, Marchou B, Lemozy J, et al. Successful treatment of *Actinobacillus actinomycetemcomitans* endocarditis with ofloxacin. Clin Microbiol Infect 2000;6:55–56.

180. Hoeprich PD. Clinical use of amphotericin B and derivatives: lore, mystique and fact. Clin Infect Dis 1992;14(Suppl 1):S114–119.

CHAPTER 7

Cardiac Surgery in Infective Endocarditis

In many patients with IE, the infection can be cured with medical treatment alone [1]. However, in 25–30% medical treatment alone is insufficient and must be combined with surgery. The purpose of surgery is to control infection by debridement and removal of necrotic tissue and to restore cardiac morphology by surgical repair and/or valve replacement. The indications and optimal timing for surgery in infective endocarditis have been recently discussed in the literature [2].

INDICATIONS

Surgery is indicated in patients with life-threatening congestive heart failure or cardiogenic shock due to surgically treatable valvular heart disease—such as severe aortic or mitral regurgitation [3] (Figure 7.1). Aortic valve cusp perforation and even leaflet dehiscence leads to severe aortic regurgitation and necessitates urgent aortic valve replacement (Figures 7.2–7.4). This applies to cases with or without proven IE if the patient has reasonable prospects of recovery and a satisfactory quality of life after surgery. Development of cardiac failure carries a mortality of >50% in patients with IE managed with only medical treatment [1]. Many studies have indicated that surgical intervention improves the prognosis of IE over medical therapy alone (10–35% versus 55–85%) [4] and a high early surgery rate is associated with good long-term results and no increase in hospital mortality [5–10]. However, randomized trials of medical versus surgical treatment do not exist and the conclusions that have emerged are often only supported by case studies. Surgery should be postponed or avoided if serious complications make the prospect of recovery unlikely.

The indications for surgery for IE in patients with stable hemodynamics are less clear and depend also on whether native or prosthetic valves are involved. Early consultation with a cardiac surgeon is advisable in case surgery is suddenly required. Surgery is indicated in patients with valvular obstruction or dehiscence, annular or aortic abscesses, pseudoaneurysms, fistulous communications, those with fungal endocarditis, those with PVE, and those with infections resistant to antibiotics (Figures 7.5–7.7). Indeed, persisting fever often represents abscess of the valve ring and surrounding structures or widespread tissue destruction and generally necessitates surgical intervention including radical debridement and sometimes extensive reconstruction [11–13]. Periannular extension occurs in 10–40% of all native valve IE and complicates aortic IE more commonly than mitral or tricuspid IE [14–16]. It occurs in 56–100% of patients with PVE [17] (Figure 7.6).

However, it should be remembered that penicillin hypersensitivity is a common cause of recurrent fever, with rash and eosinophilia being such indications. Neutropenia and impaired renal function may suggest toxic overdosing. In this case the fever usually promptly disappears after drug withdrawal. The emergence of antibiotic resistance in the infecting organism is seldom a cause and if the bacteria have been cultured and the patient given appropriate bactericidal antibiotics, then the temptation to change the treatment should be resisted.

Patients with a vegetation of diameter >10 mm have a significantly higher incidence of embolization than those with smaller vegetations [18] and the risk is higher in mitral

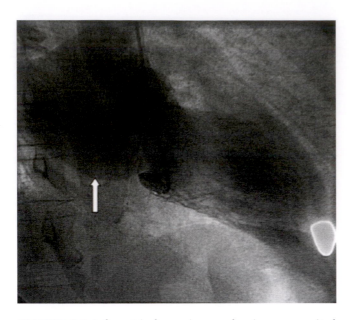

FIGURE 7.1 Left ventricular angiogram showing severe mitral regurgitation into left atrium (arrow) in a patient with endocarditis of the mitral valve.

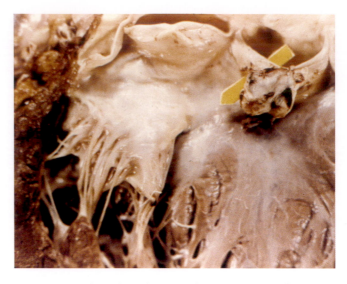

FIGURE 7.3a) Perforated aortic valve cusp due to infective endocarditis resulting in severe aortic regurgitation, heart failure, and death.

(25%) than in aortic (10%) endocarditis and especially when the anterior leaflet of the mitral valve is involved. However, surgery on the basis of vegetation size alone is controversial. Valvular vegetations can be identified and sized by echocardiography (Figure 7.8) and especially TEE. Early surgery should be considered for aortic/mitral kissing vegetations, markedly mobile vegetations, and vegetations that appear to be rapidly increasing in size (Figures 7.9–7.16).

Prior systemic embolization, recurrent emboli, persistent vegetation after a major systemic embolus, and

association with a perivalvular abscess are usually indications for surgery. This is especially so in patients who have endocarditis caused by *Staphylococcus aureus*, fungi, or *Haemophilus* spp.

Many of the important issues concerning the surgical management of PVE have been the subject of discussions and review articles [19–27]. Acute valvular regurgitation with pulmonary edema, dehiscence of a prosthetic valve, and abscess formation are absolute indications for surgery

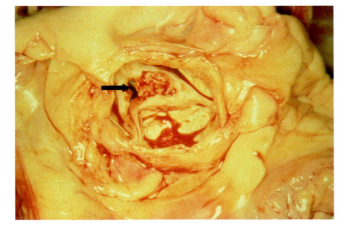

FIGURE 7.2 Vegetation on aortic valve resulting in a perforation of a valve cusp (arrow) and severe aortic regurgitation in a patient with *Staphylococcus aureus* infective endocarditis.

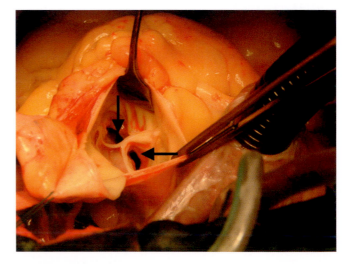

FIGURE 7.3b) Large perforations (arrows) in two cusps of the aortic valve following infective endocarditis resulted in severe aortic regurgitation and intractable heart failure. This patient successfully underwent emergency aortic valve replacement. Courtesy of Mr. N Mediratta.

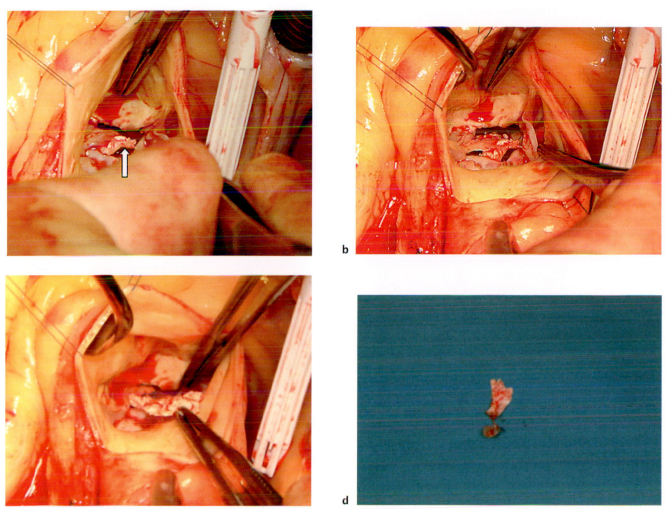

FIGURE 7.4 (**a** and **b**) This flail leaflet (arrow) on the aortic valve gives rise to severe aortic regurgitation. It was freely mobile into and out of the left ventricular outflow tract and visualized by echocardiography. (**c**) The torn, flail, and calcified leaflet is lifted by forceps. (**d**) Flail aortic valve leaflet and attached vegetation removed from patient undergoing emergency aortic valve replacement for severe aortic regurgitation. Courtesy of Mr Walid Dihmis.

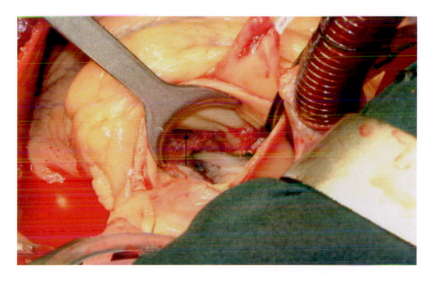

FIGURE 7.5 Aortic valve endocarditis associated with a sinus of Valsalva aneurysm. The entrance to the aneurysm is shown by the arrow.

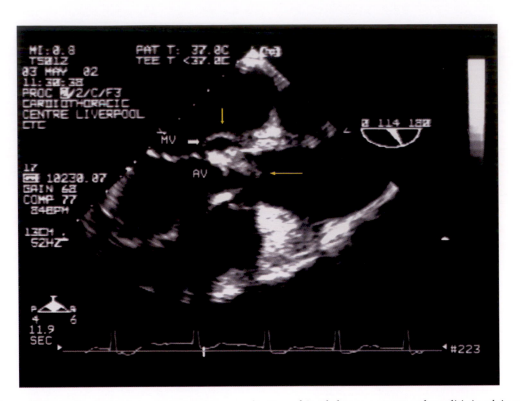

FIGURE 7.6 Paravalvular aortic abscess is a not uncommon complication of *Staphylococcus aureus* endocarditis involving the aortic valve. This TEE shows a large vegetation on a bioprosthetic aortic valve (arrow) infected by coagulase-negative *Staphylococcus*. A large paravalvular abscess is clearly visible (twin arrows). MV, mitral valve; AV, aortic valve.

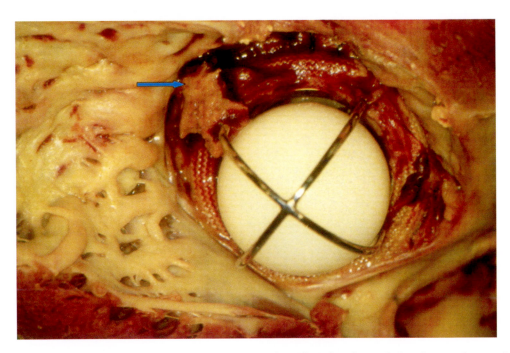

FIGURE 7.7 Starr–Edwards prosthesis infected with *Staphylococcus epidermidis*. Infected granulation tissue and vegetations are seen to be adherent to the sewing ring and struts of the prosthesis (arrow).

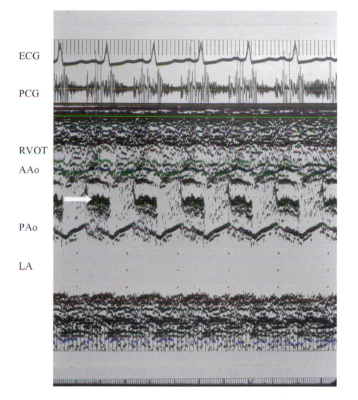

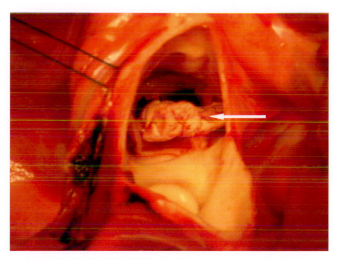

FIGURE 7.10 Large, very mobile vegetation (arrow) on aortic valve of IV drug abuser with *Staphylococcus aureus* infective endocarditis, severe aortic regurgitation, and pulmonary edema—seen at aortotomy. Figures 7.10–7.16 courtesy of Dr M. Desmond and Mr A. Rashid.

FIGURE 7.8 M-mode echocardiogram shows aortic valve vegetations (arrow). ECG, electrocardiogram; PCG, phonocardiogram; RVOT, right ventricular outflow tract; AAo, anterior aortic root wall; PAo, posterior aortic root wall; LA, left atrium.

(Figures 7.17–7.19). Patients with PVE should have their warfarin replaced by heparin in case urgent surgery is necessary. Anticoagulant therapy is potentially hazardous in patients with infective endocarditis [28].

Abdominal and splenic abscesses should be operated upon before cardiac surgery is performed.

In intravenous drug addicts with tricuspid valve endocarditis and tricuspid regurgitation, large vegetations can be treated by tricuspid valve repair, tricuspid valvectomy or vegetectomy [29–32], although valvectomy may result in permanent damage to the right ventricle, intractable right heart failure, and death. Repair has the advantage of

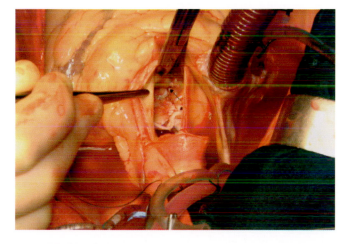

FIGURE 7.9 Fleshy vegetations (arrow) on stenotic aortic valve infected with viridans streptococci. View at aortotomy. Courtesy of Mr N. Mediratta.

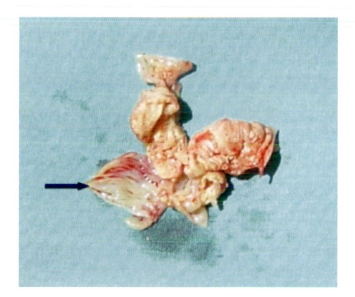

FIGURE 7.11 Large vegetations are attached to two cusps of this resected aortic valve. The arrow points to the cusp that appears free of vegetations.

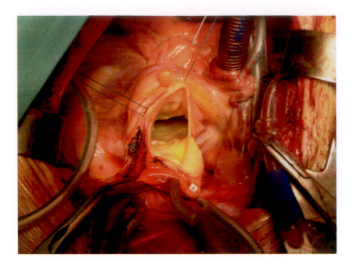

FIGURE 7.12 Infected aortic valve and vegetation removed in preparation for aortic valve implantation.

avoiding or minimizing the implantation of foreign material in the infected area while preserving tricuspid valve function. Several different techniques have been used, including cusp resection (rendering the valve bicuspid), commissural plication, the use of artificial chordae, and pericardial patch repair of the tricuspid leaflet. If tricuspid valve replacement is unavoidable, cryopreserved mitral homografts in addition to a tricuspid ring for annular stability should be considered.

Infected pacemaker electrodes may be associated with infection or abscess formation on the tricuspid valve with which it is in contact. The electrode(s) and generator have to be removed surgically (Figures 7.20–7.22).

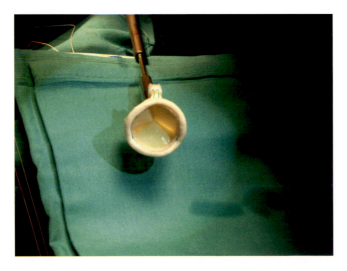

FIGURE 7.13 This Perimount tissue-valve prosthesis is selected for aortic valve replacement.

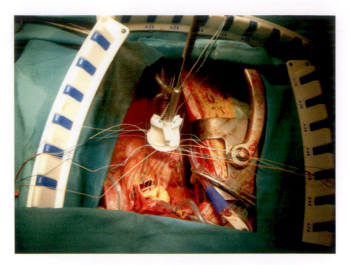

FIGURE 7.14 Prosthesis being sutured in place (1).

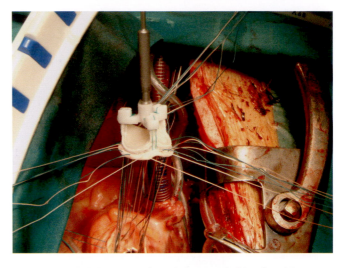

FIGURE 7.15 Prosthesis being sutured in place (2).

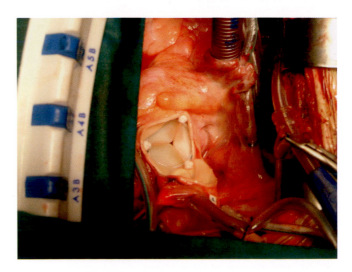

FIGURE 7.16 Aortic valve prosthesis in situ.

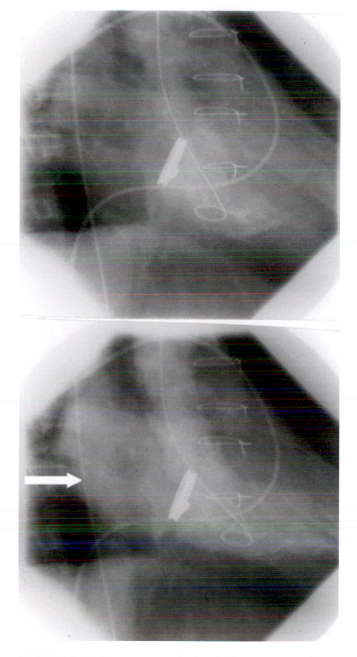

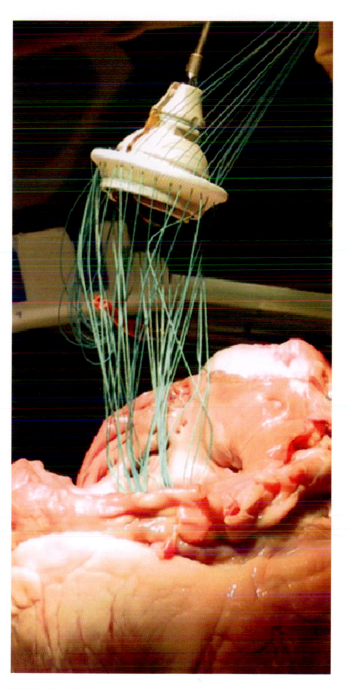

FIGURE 7.17 Severe paraprosthetic mitral regurgitation due to dehiscence of the mitral valve prosthesis caused by infective endocarditis with *Staphylococcus aureus*. This left ventricular angiogram shows contrast regurgitation into the left atrium (arrow).

FIGURE 7.18 Aortic valve replacement with a prosthetic, mechanical valve is often necessary when the native aortic valve is destroyed by infective endocarditis. This ATS® carbon bileaflet aortic valve prosthesis is about to be inserted on its holder. Courtesy of Mr M. Pullan.

Infection with certain organisms (e.g. fungi, *Coxiella burnetii*, and enterococci for which there is no synergistic bactericidal combination) rarely responds to medical treatment alone and usually requires surgery.

Intraoperative TEE may provide useful information on the exact location and extent of the infection and in the planning of surgery.

TIMING OF SURGERY

If there is an adequate indication for early surgery in the course of active IE such as severe aortic regurgitation and progressive pulmonary edema, there is little evidence that

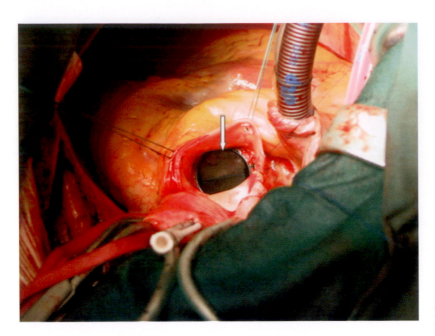

FIGURE 7.19 Bileaflet aortic valve prosthesis in place (arrow).

there is anything to be gained by delaying surgery for prolonged periods of antibiotics [4,33–35]. The frequency of early relapse and/or infection of the prosthesis after surgery is low [36,37]. If heart failure regresses, the optimal timing remains controversial, although 2 weeks of antibiotic therapy is generally considered ideal [38].

Early surgery for PVE may reduce mortality even when the period of preoperative antibiotic treatment has been brief [39,40]. Although 10 days of antibiotic therapy prior to surgery is desirable, surgery should not be delayed as postoperative endocarditis is surprisingly uncommon [41,42].

The optimal timing of surgery after a cerebral embolism is often unclear because heparinization during bypass may exacerbate the clinical course of a recent cerebral infarction [43,44]. Ideally, 10 days should be allowed to elapse in patients who have sustained a cerebral infarct, although surgical results are good within the first 72 hours [43,45–47]. Such emergency surgery may be required if IE is complicated by severe prosthetic valve dysfunction, paravalvular leaks, persistent positive blood cultures, abscesses, large vegetations, or conduction defects (Figure 7.23). At least 3 weeks should be allowed to elapse in those who have had an intracranial hemorrhage [44].

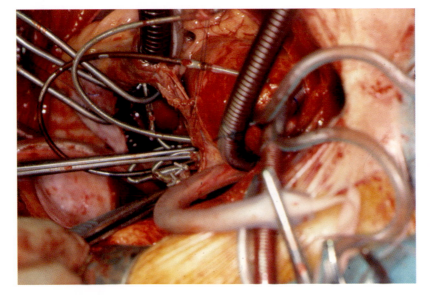

FIGURE 7.20 A 60-year-old man developed anorexia, night sweats, and weight loss 18 months after pacemaker implantation. Although he had no signs of pacemaker generator infection, blood cultures yielded *Staphylococcus epidermidis* and a vegetation could be seen on the ventricular lead by TEE. His aortic valve prosthesis showed no evidence of vegetations on echocardiography. Five weeks of IV antibiotics did not improve matters and surgical removal of the whole pacing system was performed.

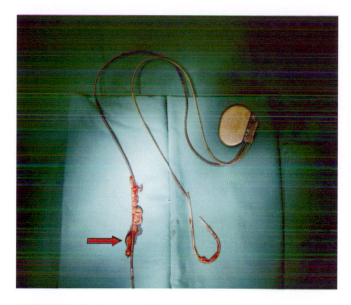

FIGURE 7.21 Removal of the whole pacing system demonstrated the large infected vegetation (arrow) which was adherent to the ventricular electrode and tricuspid valve. Courtesy of Mr A. Rashid.

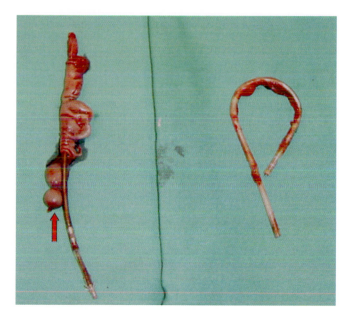

FIGURE 7.22 This vegetation (arrow) could be seen to be mobile on the transthoracic echocardiogram.

CAT and MRI scanning should be performed prior to any possible surgery in order to exclude cerebral hemorrhage [48,49]. Contemporary approaches to the management of neurosurgical complications of IE have been recently presented in the literature [50–52].

The indications for surgery for NVE and PVE are shown in Table 7.1 [53–57]. Whether antibiotic impregnation of heart valve sewing rings prevents endocarditis or is useful in the surgical treatment of endocarditis remains unclear at present [58].

RESULTS OF SURGERY

Operative mortality varies from 4% to 30%. The highest risk and poorest outcome appears to be in patients with heart failure, perivalvular abscess or aortic root abscess, as well as those with infections due to certain Gram-negative aerobic bacilli (*Escherichia coli*, *Serratia* spp., *Pseudomonas aeruginosa*), fungi, *S. aureus* and *S. epidermidis* which are resistant to penicillin and sometimes methicillin [3,14, 59,60]. Early surgical intervention is required in many

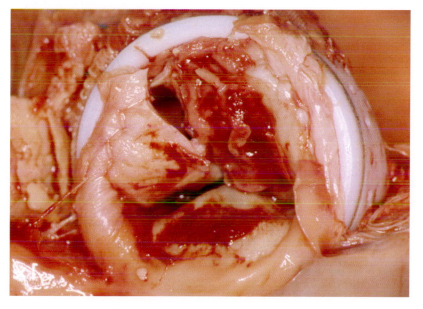

FIGURE 7.23 This bioprosthesis was totally destroyed and made severely regurgitant as a result of *Staphylococcus* endocarditis.

TABLE 7.1 Indications for surgery for native and prosthetic valve endocarditis

Native
Acute aortic regurgitation (AR) or mitral regurgitation (MR) with heart failure [86–88]
Acute AR with tachycardia and early closure of the mitral valve
Fungal endocarditis [89–94]
Annular or aortic abscess, true aneurysm of the sinus of Valsalva, true or false aneurysm of the aorta [86,87]
Evidence of valvular dysfunction and persistent infection after a prolonged period (7–10 days) of appropriate antibiotics, as indicated by
  presence of fever, leukocytosis, or bacteremia—assuming that there are no noncardiac causes for infection [86,87]
Recurrent emboli after appropriate antibiotic therapy [86,87]
Mobile vegetations >10 mm diameter
Early infection of the mitral valve—that can be repaired
Persistent pyrexia and leukocytosis with negative blood cultures [86,87]
Infection with Gram-negative organisms or organisms with a poor response to antibiotics [86,87,95]
Relapse after an adequate course of antibiotics

Prosthetic
Early prosthetic valve endocarditis (<2 months) [86,87,95]
Heart failure with prosthetic valve dysfunction
Fungal endocarditis [89,95]
Staphylococcal endocarditis unresponsive to antibiotics [86,87,95,96]
Paravalvular leak, annular or aortic root abscess [86,87,95,96]
Infection with Gram-negative organisms or organisms with a poor response to antibiotics [86,87,95]
Sinus or aortic true/false aneurysm, fistula formation
Persistent bacteremia after 7–10 days of antibiotics
Recurrent peripheral embolus
Vegetation on prosthesis
New-onset conduction disturbance
Relapse after an adequate course of antibiotics

cases but the mortality may still be >20% [61]. Among patients who have NVE, survival ranges from 70% to 80% at 5 years, although it is less optimistic in those with PVE, where surgical treatment is generally better than medical therapy alone [62]. A relapse rate of IE of 5–10% occurs when surgery is performed in the acute phase of the disease, and paravalvular regurgitation occurs in 5–15% of cases. Long-term results of surgical treatment of active infective aortic valve endocarditis with associated periannular abscess have been recently presented [63,64]. Permanent pacemaker implantation is not infrequently indicated postoperatively in patients with aortic valve endocarditis and root abscesses and temporary endocardial or epicardial leads should be in place until a permanent system is implanted (Figures 7.24–7.26).

Surgical intervention for IE in infancy and childhood and in intravenous drug abusers has been described in the literature [65,66].

Whether surgery using homograft or mechanical prostheses is best in the short or long term remains debatable and randomized trials would be necessary to settle this issue [67–85] (Figures 7.27 and 7.28). A perforation in a valve cusp or leaflet can be repaired with a pericardial patch, and kissing vegetations may be removed and

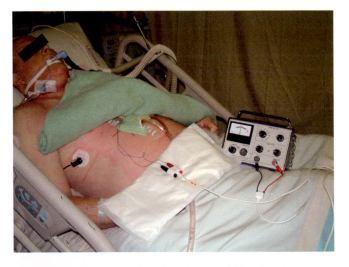

FIGURE 7.25 Epicardial pacing wires should be placed postoperatively in patients with any conduction defect as a result of infective endocarditis. They are frequently required in patients with aortic valve endocarditis and paravalvular abscess.

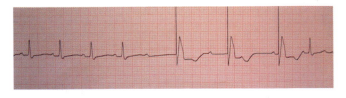

FIGURE 7.24 Pacing is frequently necessary in aortic valve endocarditis complicated by aortic root abscess.

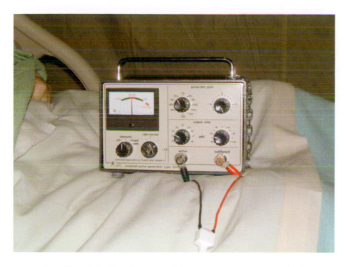

FIGURE 7.26 Pacing box used for temporary epicardial pacing after surgical intervention for infective endocarditis.

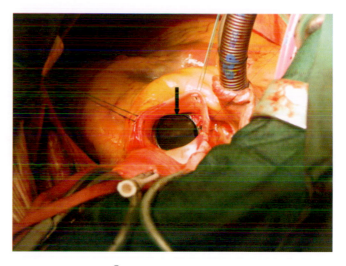

FIGURE 7.28 ATS® bileaflet mechanical valve (arrow) used for aortic valve replacement in infective endocarditis will require long-term oral anticoagulant therapy. Courtesy of Mr M. Pullan.

the valve similarly repaired. Subannular, annular, and supra-annular defects may be repaired by autologous pericardium but all abscesses must be drained and the cavity debrided. Allograft aortic root replacement is a valuable technique in the complex setting of PVE with involvement of the periannular region [74,83].

After surgery, antibiotics should be continued—the duration depends on the length of treatment preopera-tively, the susceptibility of the organism to antibiotics, the presence of paravalvular lesions, and the culture status of vegetations or valve removed.

Generally, treatment should be continued for 2 weeks postoperatively. However, when intracardiac fungal masses and vegetations persist despite antifungal therapy and surgical removal is necessary, oral medication should be prolonged postoperatively (Figure 7.29).

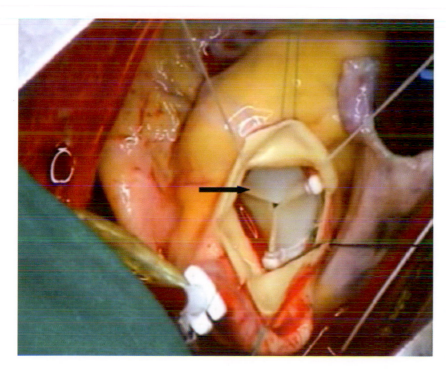

FIGURE 7.27 A Carpentier-Edwards Perimount bioprosthesis (arrow) is placed in the aortic position after removal of an infected, regurgitant mechanical prosthesis. Courtesy of Dr M. Desmond and Mr B. Fabri.

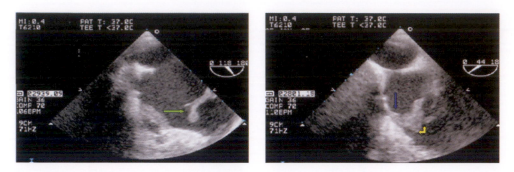

FIGURE 7.29a) Transoesophageal echocardiogram from a 48-year-old woman receiving chemotherapy with epirubicin (via a Hickman line) for breast cancer following mastectomy and axillary clearance. She developed neutropenic septicaemia due to *Candida tropicalis*. The echocardiogram (right) showed a large (20mm) vegetation (double arrow) on the anterior tricuspid valve leaflet (arrow), moderate tricuspid regurgitation and (left) a large pedunculated mobile mass (25mm long) (arrow) attached to the superior vena cava and floating in the right atrium. Courtesy of Dr. Chris Bellamy.

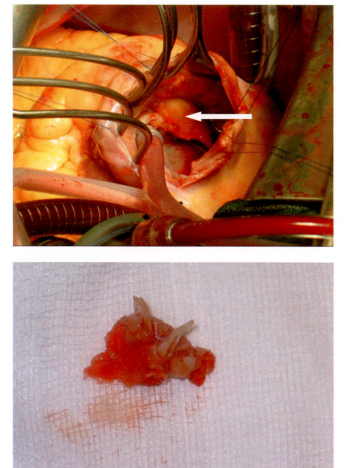

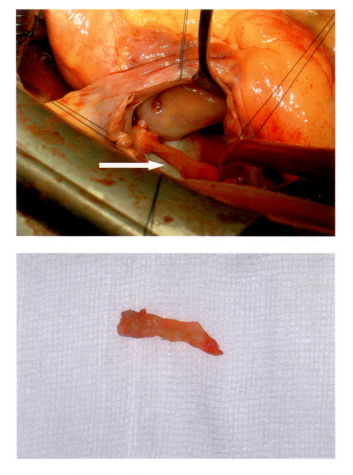

FIGURE 7.29b) Open heart surgery was necessary to remove the mass from the SVC (arrow).

FIGURE 7.29c) The tricuspid valve and its large vegetation (arrow) were also removed. The valve was replaced by a tissue valve prosthesis and the patient treated with IV amphotericin B for 4 weeks and oral voriconazole for 1 year. The large fungal mass can be seen attached to the destroyed tricuspid valve. Courtesy of Mr. A Oo.

REFERENCES

1. Verheul HA, van den Brink RB, van Vreeland T, et al. Effects of changes in management of active infective endocarditis on outcome in a 25-year period. Am J Cardiol 1993;72:682–687.

2. Delahaye F, Celard M, Roth O, de Gevigney G. Indications and optimal timing for surgery in infective endocarditis. Heart 2004;90:618–620.

3. Middlemost S, Wisenbaugh T, Meyerowitz C, et al. A case for early surgery in native left-sided endocarditis complicated by heart failure: results in 203 patients. J Am Coll Cardiol 1991;18:663–667.

4. Olaison L, Pettersson G. Current best practices and guidelines indications for surgical intervention in infective endocarditis. Infect Dis Clin North Am 2002;16:453–475.

5. Bogers AJJC, van Vreeswijk H, Verbaan CJ, et al. Early surgery for active infective endocarditis improves early and late results. Thorac Cardiovasc Surg 1991;39:284–287.

6. Jubair KA, Al Fagih MR, Ashmeg A, et al. Cardiac operations during active endocarditis. J Thorac Cardiovasc Surg 1992;104:487–490.

7. Vlessis AA, Hovaguimian H, Jaggers J, et al. Infective endocarditis: ten-year review of medical and surgical therapy. Ann Thorac Surg 1996;61:1217–1222.

8. Dehler S, Elert O. Early and late prognosis following valve replacement for bacterial endocarditis of the native valve. Thorac Cardiovasc Surg 1995;43:83–89.

9. Castillo JC, Anguita MP, Ramirez A, et al. Long-term outcome of infective endocarditis in patients who were not drug addicts: a 10 year study. Heart 2000;83:525–530.

10. Alexiou C, Langley SM, Stafford H, et al. Surgery for active culture-positive endocarditis: determinants of early and late outcomes. Ann Thorac Surg 2000;69:1448–1454.

11. Douglas A, Moore-Gillon J, Eykyn SJ. Fever during treatment of infective endocarditis. Lancet 1986;i:1341–1343.

12. Graupner C, Vilacosta I, SanRoman J, et al. Periannular extension of infective endocarditis. J Am Coll Cardiol 2002;39:1204–1211.

13. Choussat R, Thomas D, Isnard R, et al. Perivalvular abscess associated with endocarditis: clinical features and prognostic factors of overall success in a series of 233 cases. Perivalvular Abscess French Multicentre Study. Eur Heart J 1999;20:232–241.

14. Stinson EB. Surgical treatment of infective endocarditis. Prog Cardiovasc Dis 1979;22:145–168.

15. Becher H, Hanrath P, Bleifeld W, Bleese N. Correlation of echocardiographic and surgical findings in acute bacterial endocarditis. Eur Heart J 1984;5(Suppl C):67–70.

16. Arnett EN, Roberts WC. Prosthetic valve endocarditis: clinicopathologic analysis of 22 necropsy patients with comparison of observations in 74 necropsy patients with active endocarditis involving natural left-sided cardiac valves. Am J Cardiol 1976;38:281–292.

17. Blumberg EA, Karalis DA, Chandrasekaran K, et al. Endocarditis-associated paravalvular abscesses: do clinical parameters predict the presence of abscess? Chest 1995;107:898–903.

18. Scarvelis D, Malcolm I. Embolization of a huge tricuspid valve bacterial vegetation. J Am Soc Echocardiogr 2002;15:185–187.

19. Stewart WJ, Shan K. The diagnosis of prosthetic valve endocarditis by echocardiography. Semin Thorac Cardiovasc Surg 1995;7:7–12.

20. Ergin MA. Surgical techniques in prosthetic valve endocarditis. Semin Thorac Cardiovasc Surg 1995;7:54–60.

21. David TE. The surgical treatment of patients with prosthetic valve endocarditis. Semin Thorac Cardiovasc Surg 1995;7:47–53.

22. Joyce F, Tingleff J, Pettersson G. The Ross operation in the treatment of prosthetic aortic valve endocarditis. Semin Thorac Cardiovasc Surg 1995;7:38–46.

23. Camacho MT, Cosgrove DM 3rd. Homografts in the treatment of prosthetic valve endocarditis. Semin Thorac Cardiovasc Surg 1995;7:32–37.

24. McGiffin DC, Kirklin JK. The impact of aortic valve homografts on the treatment of aortic prosthetic valve endocarditis. Semin Thorac Cardiovasc Surg 1995;7:25–31.

25. Gordon SM, Keys TF. Bloodstream infections in patients with implanted prosthetic cardiac valves. Semin Thorac Cardiovasc Surg 1995;7:2–6.

26. Lytle BW. Surgical treatment of prosthetic valve endocarditis. Semin Thorac Cardiovasc Surg 1995;7:13–19.

27. Lytle BW. Prosthetic valve endocarditis. Introduction. Semin Thorac Cardiovasc Surg 1995;7:1.

28. Tornos P, Alnurante B, Mirabet S. Infective endocarditis due to *Staphylococcus aureus*: deleterious effect of anticoagulant therapy. Arch Intern Med 1999;159:473–475.

29. Nihoyannopoulos P. Tricuspid valvectomy following tricuspid valve endocarditis in an intravenous drug addict. Heart 2001;86:144.

30. Carozza A, Penzulli A, De Feo M, et al. Tricuspid repair for infective endocarditis: clinical and echocardiographic results. Tex Heart Inst J 2001;28:96–101.

31. Yee ES, Khonsari S. Right-sided infective endocarditis: valvuloplasty, valvectomy or replacement. J Cardiovasc Surg 1989;30:744–748.

32. Hughes CF, Noble N. Vegetectomy: an alternative surgical treatment for infective endocarditis of the atrioventricular valves in drug addicts. J Thorac Cardiovasc Surg 1988;95:857–861.

33. Reinhartz O, Herrmann M, Redling F, Zerkowski HR. Timing of surgery in patients with acute infective endocarditis. J Cardiovasc Surg 1996;37:397–400.

34. Wilson WR, Davidson GK, Giuliani ER, et al. Cardiac valve replacement in congestive heart failure due to infective endocarditis. Mayo Clin Proc 1979;54:223–226.

35. Moon MR, Stinson EB, Miller DC. Surgical treatment of endocarditis. Prog Cardiovasc Dis 1997;40:239–264.

36. Karchmer AW, Stinson EB. The role of surgery in infective endocarditis. In: Remington JS, Schwartz MN, eds. Current Clinical Topics in Infectious Diseases. New York: McGraw-Hill; 1980:124–157.

37. Jung JY, Saab SB, Almond CH. The case for early surgical treatment of left-sided primary infective endocarditis: a collective review. J Thorac Cardiovasc Surg 1975;70:509–518.

38. Acar J, Michel PL, Varenne O, Michaud P, Rafik T. Surgical treatment of infective endocarditis. Eur Heart J 1995;16(Suppl B):94–98.

39. Saffle JR, Gardner P, Schoenbaum SC, Wild W. Prosthetic valve endocarditis: the case for prompt valve replacement. J Thorac Cardiovasc Surg 1977;73:416–420.

40. Peri CM, Vuk F, Huski CR. Active infective endocarditis: low mortality associated with early surgical treatment. Cardiovasc Surg 2000;8:208–213.

41. Karchmer AW. Treatment of prosthetic valve endocarditis. In: Sand MA, Kaye D, Root RT, eds. Endocarditis. New York: Churchill Livingstone; 1984.

42. Richardson JV, Karp RB, Kirklin JW, Dismukes WE. Treatment of infective endocarditis: a 10 year comparative analysis. Circulation 1978;58:589–597.

43. Parrino PE, Kron IL, Ross SD, et al. Does a focal neurological deficit contraindicate operation in a patient with endocarditis? Ann Thorac Surg 1999;67:59–64.

44. Gillinov AM, Shah RV, Curtis WE, et al. Valve replacement in patients with endocarditis and acute neurologic deficit. Ann Thorac Surg 1996;61:1125–1129.

45. Eishi K, Kawazoe K, Kuriyama Y, et al. Surgical management of infective endocarditis associated with cerebral complications. Multi-center retrospective study in Japan. J Thorac Cardiovasc Surg 1995;110:1745–1755.

46. Ting W, Silverman N, Levitsky S. Valve replacement in patients with endocarditis and cerebral septic embolism. Ann Thorac Surg 1991;51:18–21.

47. Piper C, Wiemer M, Schulte HG, Horstkotte D. Stroke is not a contraindication for urgent valve replacement in acute infective endocarditis. J Heart Valve Dis 2001;10:703–711.

48. Vilacosta I, Gomez J. Complementary role of MRI in infectious endocarditis. Echocardiography 1995;12:673–676.

49. Bertorini TE, Laster RE Jr, Thompson BF, Gelfand M. Magnetic resonance imaging of the brain in bacterial endocarditis. Arch Intern Med 1989;149:815–817.

50. Turtz AR, Yocom SS. Contemporary approaches to the management of neurosurgical complications of infective endocarditis. Curr Infect Dis Rep 2001;3:337–346.

51. Utoh J, Miyauchi Y, Goto H, et al. Endovascular approach for an intracranial mycotic aneurysm associated with infective endocarditis. J Thorac Cardiovasc Surg 1995;110:557–559.

52. Salgado AV, Furlan AJ, Keys TF. Mycotic aneurysm, subarachnoid hemorrhage, and indications for cerebral angiography in infective endocarditis. Stroke 1987;18:1057–1060.

53. Dodge A, Hurni M, Ruchat P, et al. Surgery in native valve endocarditis: indications, results and risk factors. Eur J Cardiothorac Surg 1995;9:330–334.

54. Aranki SF, Santini F, Adams DH, et al. Aortic valve endocarditis. Determinants of early survival and late morbidity. Circulation 1994;90(Suppl II):175–182.

55. Olaison L, Hogevik H, Myken P, et al. Early surgery in infective endocarditis. QJM 1996;89:267–278.

56. Reinhartz O, Herrmann M, Redling F, et al. Timing of surgery in patients with acute infective endocarditis. J Cardiovasc Surg 1996;37:397–400.

57. Lytle BW, Priest BP, Taylor PC, et al. Surgical treatment of prosthetic valve endocarditis. J Thorac Cardiovasc Surg 1996;111:198–207.

58. Cimbollek M, Nies B, Wenz R, Kreuter J. Antibiotic-impregnated heart valve sewing rings for treatment and prophylaxis of bacterial endocarditis. Antimicrob Agents Chemother 1996;40:1432–1437.

59. Mullany C, Chau Y, Schaff H, et al. Early and late survival after surgical treatment of culture-positive active endocarditis. Mayo Clin Proc 1995;70:517–525.

60. John RM, Pugsley W, Treasure T, Sturridge MF, Swanton RH. Aortic root complications of infective endocarditis. Influence on surgical outcome. Eur Heart J 1991;12:241–248.

61. Espersen F, Frimodt-Noller N. *Staphylococcus aureus* endocarditis. A review of 119 cases. Arch Intern Med 1986;146:1118–1121.

62. Delany D, Pellerini M, Carrier M, et al. Immediate and long-term results of valve replacement for native and prosthetic valve endocarditis. Ann Thorac Surg 2000;70:1219–1223.

63. Knosalla C, Weng Y, Yankah AC, et al. Surgical treatment of active infective aortic valve endocarditis with associated periannular abscess—11 year results. Eur Heart J 2000;21:490–497.

64. d'Udekem Y, David TE, Feindel CM, et al. Long-term results of operation for paravalvular abscess. Ann Thorac Surg 1996;62:48–53.

65. Nomura F, Penny DJ, Menahem S, et al. Surgical intervention for infective endocarditis in infancy and childhood. Ann Thorac Surg 1995;60:90–95.

66. Mathew J, Abreo G, Namburi K, et al. Results of surgical treatment for infective endocarditis in intravenous drug users. Chest 1995;108:73–77.

67. Moon MR, Miller DL, Moore KA, et al. Treatment of endocarditis with valve replacement: the question of tissue versus mechanical prosthesis. Ann Thorac Surg 2001;71:1164–1171.

68. Niwaya K, Knott-Craig CJ, Santangelo K, et al. Advantage of autograft and homograft valve replacement for complex aortic valve endocarditis. Ann Thorac Surg 1999;67:1603–1608.

69. Grandmougin D, Prat A, Fayad G, et al. Acute aortic endocarditis with annular destruction: assessment of surgical treatment with cryopreserved valvular homografts. J Heart Valve Dis 1999;8:234–241.

70. Haydock D, Barratt-Boyes B, Macedo T, et al. Aortic valve replacement for active infectious endocarditis in 108 patients. A

comparison of freehand allograft valves with mechanical prostheses and bioprostheses. J Thorac Cardiovasc Surg 1992;103: 130–139.

71. Petrou M, Wong K, Albertucci M, et al. Evaluation of unstented aortic homografts for the treatment of prosthetic aortic valve endocarditis. Circulation 1994;90(part 2):198–204.

72. Zwischenberger JB, Shalaby TZ, Conti VR. Viable cryopreserved aortic homograft for aortic valve endocarditis and annular abscesses. Ann Thorac Surg 1989;48:365–370.

73. Pagano D, Allen SM, Bonser RS. Homograft aortic valve and root replacement for severe destructive native or prosthetic endocarditis. Eur J Cardiothorac Surg 1994;8:173–176.

74. Dossche KM, Defauw JJ, Ernst SM, et al. Allograft aortic root replacement in prosthetic aortic valve endocarditis: a review of 32 patients. Ann Thorac Surg 1997;63:1644–1649.

75. O'Brien MF, Stafford EG, Gardner MA, et al. A comparison of aortic valve replacement with viable cryopreserved and fresh allograft valves, with a note on chromosomal studies. J Thorac Cardiovasc Surg 1987;94:812–823.

76. McGiffin DC, Galbraith AJ, McLachlan GL, et al. Aortic valve infection. Risk factors for death and recurrent endocarditis after aortic valve replacement. J Thorac Cardiovasc Surg 1992;104: 511–520.

77. Dearani JA, Orszulak TA, Schaff HV, et al. Results of allograft aortic valve replacement for complex endocarditis. J Thorac Cardiovasc Surg 1997;113:285–291.

78. Edwards MB, Ratnatunga CP, Dore CJ, et al. Thirty-day mortality and long-term survival following surgery for prosthetic endocarditis: a study from the UK heart valve registry. Eur J Cardiothorac Surg 1998;14:156–164.

79. D'Udekem Y, David TE, Feindel CM, et al. Long-term results of surgery for active infective endocarditis. Eur J Cardiothorac Surg 1997;11:46–52.

80. Jault F, Gandjbakhch I, Rama A, et al. Active native valve endocarditis: determinants of operative death and late mortality. Ann Thorac Surg 1997;63:1737–1741.

81. Ladowski JS, Deschner WP. Allograft replacement of the aortic valve for active endocarditis. J Cardiovasc Surg 1996;37(Suppl 1):61–62.

82. Wos S, Jasinski M, Bachowski R. Results of mechanical prosthetic valve replacement in active valvular endocarditis. J Cardiovasc Surg 1996;37(Suppl 1):29–32.

83. Robicsek F. Are allografts the "choice" in infectious endocarditis with periannular abscess? Eur Heart J 2000;21:421.

84. Yankah AC, Klose H, Petzina R, et al. Surgical management of acute aortic root endocarditis with valve homograft: 13 year experience. Eur J Cardiovasc Surg 2002;21:260–267.

85. Guerra JM, Tornos MP, Permanye-Miralda G, et al. Long-term results of mechanical prostheses for treatment of active endocarditis. Heart 2001;86:63–68.

86. Durack DT. Infective endocarditis. In: Schlant R, Hurst WJ, eds. The Heart, 7th edn companion handbook. New York: McGraw Hill; 1990:153–167.

87. Scheld WM, Sande MA. Endocarditis and intravascular infections. In: Mandell GL, Douglas RG Jr, Dolin R, eds. Principles and Practice of Infectious Diseases, 4th edn. New York: Churchill Livingstone, 1995:740–783.

88. Bayer AS, Bolger AF, Taubert KA, et al. Diagnosis and management of infective endocarditis and its complications. Circulation 1998;98:2936–2948.

89. Guzman F, Cartmill I, Holden MP, Freeman R. *Candida* endocarditis: report of four cases. Int J Cardiol 1987;16:131–136.

90. Woods GL, Wood P, Shaw BW Jr. *Aspergillus* endocarditis in patients without prior cardiovascular surgery: report of a case in a liver transplant recipient and review. Rev Infect Dis 1989;11:263–272.

91. Fowler VG, Durack DT. Infective endocarditis. Curr Opin Cardiol 1994;9:389–400.

92. Kawamoto T, Nakano S, Matsuda H, et al. *Candida* endocarditis with saddle embolism: a successful surgical intervention. Ann Thorac Surg 1989;48:723–724.

93. Tanka M, Toshio A, Hosokawa S, et al. Tricuspid valve *Candida* endocarditis cured by valve-sparing debridement. Ann Thorac Surg 1989;48:857–858.

94. Isalska BJ, Stanbridge TN. Fluconazole in the treatment of candidal prosthetic valve endocarditis. BMJ 1988;297:178–179.

95. Douglas JL, Cobbs CG. Prosthetic valve endocarditis. In: Kaye D, ed. Infective Endocarditis, 2nd edn. New York: Raven Press; 1992:375–396.

96. Tucker KJ, Johnson JA, Ong T, et al. Medical management of prosthetic aortic valve endocarditis and aortic root abscess. Am Heart J 1993;125:1195–1197.

CHAPTER 8

Prognosis

The determinants of early and late survival in patients with IE have been identified [1]. Several factors worsen the prognosis of IE and early surgical intervention may be necessary [2].

Clinical factors include old age, the presence of heart failure, renal failure, neurological symptoms, systemic emboli, and delay in diagnosis. Persistent fever beyond the first week of treatment often indicates the development of complications such as progressive valve destruction, extension of infection to the valve's annulus, development of perivalvular abscess, or the presence of septic emboli.

Bacteriological factors include the causative organism, with a worse prognosis in the case of *Staphylococcus aureus*, certain Gram-negative aerobic bacilli, and fungi. These often present as acute IE and produce severe intracardiac destruction and major embolic complications. Early surgical intervention is frequently required and the mortality rate is >20% [3].

Echocardiographic factors include aortic valve endocarditis, PVE, and ring abscesses when persisting infection is more likely and surgery often inevitable [4]. The presence of recent, large (> 10 mm), very mobile, pedunculated vegetations increases the risk of systemic embolization, which may significantly affect prognosis.

The cure rate for NVE is >90% for streptococci, 75–90% for enterococci, and 60–75% for *S. aureus* [5–8]. The usual causes of death are heart failure, emboli, rupture of mycotic aneurysms, postoperative complications, renal failure, and overwhelming infection. The prognosis is worse in PVE than in NVE, and on rare occasions only heart transplantation can resolve intractable infection on prosthetic valves [9]. Late prosthetic valve endocarditis has a better prognosis than early prosthetic valve endocarditis, with mortality rates of 19–50% and 41–80% respectively [10–15]. Valvular dysfunction, dehiscence, and intracardiac abscesses are commoner in early infection and the antibiotic-resistant organisms associated with early disease contribute to the higher mortality.

In 1995, Delahaye et al reported on the long-term prognosis of IE [16]. In their series (1970–1986), global survival was 75% at 6 months and 57% at 5 years, with the annual instantaneous risk of death being 0.55 at 6 months, 0.18 at 1 year, then 0.03. After 1 year, the only factor influencing prognosis was age. The risk of recurrence appears to be 0.3–2.5/100 patient-years [16,17].

Castillo et al (1987–1997) reported a 5-year survival of 71% [18]. In NVE, 5-year survival has been reported to be 88–96%, in contrast to PVE where 5-year survival rate is 60–82% [18–20]. Late PVE may have 5-year survival rates of 80–82% [18,21].

Netzer et al [22] reported that long-term survival following IE is 50% after 10 years and is predicted by early surgical treatment, age <55 years, lack of congestive heart failure, and the initial presence of more symptoms of IE.

The long-term results of multivalvular surgery for IE have been recently reported [23].

REFERENCES

1. Aranki SF, Adams DH, Rizzo RJ, et al. Determinants of early mortality and late survival in mitral valve endocarditis. Circulation 1995;92:143–149.

2. Mansur AJ, Grinberg M, Cardoso RH, et al. Determinants of prognosis in 300 episodes of infective endocarditis. Thorac Cardiovasc Surg 1996;44:2–10.

3. Espersen F, Frimodt-Moller N. *Staphylococcus aureus* endocarditis. A review of 119 cases. Arch Intern Med 1986;146:1118–1121.

4. Rohmann S, Erbel R, Mohr-Kahaly S, Meyer J. Use of transoesophageal echocardiography in the diagnosis of abscess in infective endocarditis. Eur Heart J 1995;16(Suppl B): 54–62.

5. Bisno AL, Dismukes WE, Durack DT, et al. Antimicrobial treatment of infective endocarditis due to viridans streptococci, enterococci and staphylococci. JAMA 1989;261:1471–1477.

6. Wilson WR, Geraci JE. Treatment of streptococcal infective endocarditis. Am J Med 1985;78(Suppl 6B):128–137.

7. Faville RJ Jr, Zaske DE, Kaplan EL, et al. *Staphylococcus aureus* endocarditis: combined therapy with vancomycin and rifampicin. JAMA 1978;240:1963–1965.

8. Malquarti V, Saradarian W, Etienne J, et al. Prognosis of native valve infective endocarditis. A review of 253 cases. Eur Heart J 1984;5(Suppl C)11–20.

9. DiSesa VJ, Sloss LJ, Cohn LH. Heart transplantation for intractable prosthetic valve endocarditis. J Heart Transplant 1990;9:142–143.

10. Cowgill LD, Addonizio VP, Hopeman AR, Harken AH. Prosthetic valve endocarditis. Curr Probl Cardiol 1986;11:617–664.

11. Brottier E, Gin H, Brottier L, et al. Prosthetic valve endocarditis: diagnosis and prognosis. Eur Heart J 1984;5(Suppl C)123–127.

12. Cowgill LD, Addonizio VP, Hopeman AR, Harken AH. A practical approach to prosthetic valve endocarditis. Ann Thorac Surg 1987;43:450–457.

13. Leport C, Vilde JL, Bricaire F, et al. Fifty cases of late prosthetic valve endocarditis: improvement in prognosis over a 15 year period. Br Heart J 1987;58:66–71.

14. Dismukes WE. Prosthetic valve endocarditis. Factors influencing outcome and recommendations for therapy. In: Bisno AL, ed. Treatment of Infective Endocarditis. New York: Grune & Stratton; 1981:167–191.

15. Bayliss R, Clark C, Oakley CM, et al. Incidence, mortality and prevention of infective endocarditis. J R Coll Physicians 1986;20:15–20.

16. Delahaye F, Ecochard R, de Gevigney G, et al. The long-term prognosis of infective endocarditis. Eur Heart J 1995;16(Suppl B):48–53.

17. Renzulli A, Carozza A, Romano G, et al. Recurrent infective endocarditis: a multivariate analysis of 21 years of experience. Ann Thorac Surg 2001;72:39–43.

18. Castillo JC, Anguita MP, Ramirez A, et al. Long-term outcome of infective endocarditis in patients who were not drug addicts: a 10 year study. Heart 2000;83:525–530.

19. Tornos MP, Permanyer-Miralda G, Olona M, et al. Long term complications of native valve infective endocarditis in non addicts. Ann Intern Med 1992;117:567–572.

20. Calderwood SP, Swinsky LA, Karchmer AW, et al. Prosthetic valve endocarditis. Analysis of factors affecting outcome of therapy. J Thorac Cardiovasc Surg 1986;92:776–783.

21. Tornos P, Almirante B, Olona M, et al. Clinical outcome and long-term prognosis of late prosthetic valve endocarditis: a 20-year experience. Clin Infect Dis 1997;24:381–386.

22. Netzer ROM, Altwegg SC, Zollinger E, et al. Infective endocarditis: determinants of long term outcome. Heart 2002;88:61–66.

23. Mihaljevic T, Byrne JG, Cohn LH, Aranki SF. Long-term results of multivalvar surgery for infective multivalve endocarditis. Eur J Cardiothorac Surg 2001;20:842–846.

APPENDIX 1

Abbreviations

AICD	Automatic implantable cardioverter defibrillator	IM	Intramuscular
AIDS	Acquired immunodeficiency syndrome	IV	Intravenous
AR	Aortic regurgitation	MBC	Minimal bactericidal concentration
AS	Aortic stenosis	MIC	Minimal inhibitory concentration
ASD	Atrial septal defect	MIF	Microimmunofluorescence
ATS®	Advancing the standard	MR	Mitral regurgitation
CAT	Computer-assisted tomography	MRI	Magnetic resonance imaging
CNE	Culture-negative endocarditis	MRSA	Methicillin-resistant *Staphylococcus aureus*
CO$_2$	Carbon dioxide	NVE	Native valve endocarditis
CPB	Cardiopulmonary bypass	PAE	Post-antibiotic effect
CRP	C-reactive protein	PCG	Phonocardiogram
CSF	Cerebrospinal fluid	PCI	Percutaneous Coronary Intervention
2-D	Two-dimensional	PCR	Polymerase chain reaction
DNA	Deoxyribose nucleic acid	PDA	Patent ductus arteriosus
ECG	Electrocardiogram	PFO	Patent foramen ovale
ECHO	Echocardiography	PTCA	Percutaneous Transluminal Coronary Angioplasty
ESR	Erythrocyte sedimentation rate	PVE	Prosthetic valve endocarditis
FC	Flucytosine	spp.	Species
GA	General anesthesia	TEE	Transesophageal echocardiography
GISA	Glycopeptide intermediate resistance *Staphylococcus aureus*	TTE	Transthoracic echocardiography
		TV	Tricuspid valve
IE	Infective endocarditis	VISA	Vancomycin intermediate resistance *Staphylococcus aureus*
IgA, IgG	Immunoglobulin A, immunoglobulin G	VRE	Vancomycin-resistant enterococci

INDEX